When the Twain Meet

The Henry E. Sigerist Supplements to the
Bulletin of the History of Medicine

New Series, no. 5
Editor: Lloyd G. Stevenson

Henry E. Sigerist, recruited by William H. Welch to be director of the
Johns Hopkins Institute of the History of Medicine, was the founder of the
Bulletin of the History of Medicine and also of the first series of supplements, which extended from 1943 to 1951. It was Sigerist's resolve that the
Bulletin should provide the organ not only of the Johns Hopkins Institute
but also of the American Association, and to this day it subserves both
functions. It is therefore eminently suitable that the new series should bear
the founder's name and perpetuate his scholarly interests. These interests
were so broad and so varied that the supplements will recognize no narrow
limits in range of theme and will publish historical essays of greater scope
than the *Bulletin* itself can accommodate. It is not too much to hope that in
time the Sigerist supplements will help to extend the purview of medical
history.

Other Books in the New Series

1. *Almost Persuaded: American Physicians and Compulsory Health
Insurance, 1912-1920,* by Ronald L. Numbers, M.D.
2. *William Harvey and His Age: The Professional and Social Context of
the Discovery of the Circulation,* edited by Jerome J. Bylebyl
3. *The Clinical Training of Doctors: An Essay of 1793*
by Philippe Pinel, edited and translated, with an introductory essay, by
Dora B. Weiner
4. *Times, Places, and Persons: Aspects of the History of Epidemio –
logy,* edited by Abraham Lilienfeld, M.D.

John Z. Bowers served as president of the Josiah Macy, Jr., Foundation from 1965 to 1980. He is the author of *Medical Education in Japan, Doctors on Desima,* and *Western Medical Pioneers in Feudal Japan.*

WHEN THE TWAIN MEET

The Rise of Western Medicine in Japan

JOHN Z. BOWERS, M.D.

The Johns Hopkins University Press
Baltimore and London

The Johns Hopkins University Press, Baltimore, Maryland 21218
The Johns Hopkins Press Ltd., London

Library of Congress Cataloging in Publication Data

Bowers, John Z 1913-
    When the twain meet.

    (The Henry E. Sigerist supplements to the Bulletin
of the history of medicine; new ser., no. 5)
    Bibliography: p.
    Includes index.
    1. Medicine—Japan—History—19th century.
2. Physicians, Foreign—Japan—History—19th century.
I. Title. II. Series: Henry E. Sigerist supplements
to the Bulletin of the history of medicine; new ser.,
no. 5. [DNLM: 1. History of medicine, 19th cent.—
Japan. W1 HE896 no. 5 / WZ70 JJ3 B7wa]
R624.B68   610.952   80-22356
ISBN 0-8018-2432-X

Contents

To
Dr. Shields Warren
Whose inspiration
guided my life

Preface

During the two years, 1962-64, I spent as a visiting professor at Kyoto National University studying medical education in Japan, I became intrigued with the introduction of Western medicine to that country when it had been officially sealed off from the West for over two centuries—from 1638 to 1853. My interest was heightened by the fact that although the subject had received little attention in the West, rich resources were available in Japanese, Dutch, and German archives. Fortunately, in the course of those two years I established contacts with Japanese scholars who facilitated access to resources in their country. I also benefited from comparable contacts in Germany and the Netherlands.

After the completion of my book, *Medical Education in Japan,* published in 1965, I turned my studies to another aspect of medicine in Japan, and *Western Medical Pioneers in Feudal Japan* was published in 1969. I then began research on the official introduction of German medicine in 1870, and, as is not uncommon, I uncovered a large body of new information from the earlier peiods: it has been incorporated in this manuscript.

I am grateful to the directors of the Macy Foundation for their financial support.

The distinguished American historian on Japan, Hugh R. Borton, has graciously read every word of this manuscript and has offered numerous important suggestions.

I have benefited from the counsel and assistance of a number of other individuals: in Japan, Professors Ogawa Teizo, Otori Ranzaburo, Ogata Tomio, and Okamoto Michio. The late Professor Johannes Steudel, Dr. Toska Hesekiel, and Professor Niklaus Mani provided important German materials. My pursuit of information on the Dutch in Japan received invaluable assistance from the Reijksarchief in the Hague.

Mrs. Atsumi Minami, librarian of the historical section of the Biomedical Library, University of California Medical Center, San Francisco, made available rich resources and provided valuable assistance. Mrs. Judith Sonntag proved to be an excellent editor, and Miss Dorothy Hennessey spent many hours as my associate.

Finally, my wife, Akiko K. Bowers, has been an inestimable colleague in the preparation and completion of all aspects of the manuscript. I owe her special gratitude that I cannot adequately express.

When the Twain Meet

1

The Background

For two and a half centuries, Japan could be described as one of the most feudalistic nations in world history.[1] This situation became a reality when Tokugawa Ieyasu (1542-1616) achieved supremacy as victor in the battle of Sekigahara in 1600. Three years later, he established his capital at a castle in Edo (now Tokyo) and developed it into a massive, virtually impregnable fortress. In the same year, Ieyasu assumed his historic title, *shogun,* an abbreviation for *Seiitaishogun* ("barbarian-destroying great general"). He was determined to create an enduring political stability that he could pass on to his heirs. Essential to the achievement of this goal was the expulsion of foreigners; therefore, between 1633 and 1636 Ieyasu's grandson, Iemitsu, issued a series of decrees for a *sakoku* ("chained country"). No Japanese were permitted to leave the country, Japanese residents abroad could not return, and all foreigners were to be banished. In 1638, the construction of ships suitable for ocean voyages was banned. The Dutch alone were allowed to maintain a small factory, heavily guarded by the Japanese, on the island of Dejima ("going-out island") at Nagasaki. The emperor, now powerless, lived in his beautiful palace in Miyako, receiving material support from the Tokugawa.

Some 260 *daimyo* (feudal lords) ruled their fiefs, known as *han,* at the pleasure of the *shogun.* Those who were related to him were known as *shimpan.* A second group, and the largest number, the *fudai* (hereditary lords), had been vassals of Ieyasu before the battle of Sekigahara. They constituted the administrative and military foundation of the shogunate and occupied the central region, the Kanto plain, where they could protect the castle at Edo. A third and potentially dangerous group, the *tozama* (outer) *daimyo,* included enemies of Ieyasu or those who had been neutral at Sekigahara; they were treated with suspicion. In turn, they nursed old grudges and became the core of the opposition that led to the eventual overthrow of the Tokugawa. The *tozama* were largely relegated to the western and northern perimeters—north and west Honshu—and to the islands of Shikoku and Kyushu. The Satsuma and the Hizen on Kyushu, the Tosa on Shikoku, and the Choshu on the western extremity of Honshu

[1] The term "feudalistic" refers here to an agriculturally and militarily based society with a rigid clan structure, in which loyalty to locally powerful men was a prevailing ethos.

1

were the strongest *tozama* fiefs. The magistrates and chief ministers of the shogunate were known as the *Bakufu* ("tent government").[2]

Although they were in theory autonomous, the *daimyo* were strictly controlled by the Tokugawa in order to prevent any military plots. Special regulations set out the number of men who could bear arms, as well as the extent of fortifications. An important security measure was *sankin kotai* ("alternating in attendance"), which demanded that the wives and children of the *daimyo* reside in Edo as permanent hostages. Furthermore, most of the *daimyo* were required to spend alternate years in Edo. For this, they constructed *yashiki* (buildings and grounds); some of these would serve as compounds for the Westerners who came to Japan after the Meiji Restoration. A crucial artery was the Tokaido, which connected Sanjo Bridge in Miyako with Nihonbashi in Edo. It featured fifty-three posting stations (*seki*), immortalized by the renowned nineteenth-century artist Ando Hiroshige (1797-1858), a master of the wood-block print. Travelers were scrutinized at these stations. At the most important one, Hakonenoseki, located at the pass separating Kanto from Kansai, the government's fear was of "guns up and women down." (The phrase refers to the fact that weapons being smuggled into Edo or women hostages fleeing the city might be signs of an impending rebellion.) The Tokaido was one of the most congested thoroughfares in the world, crowded as it was with Japanese excursion parties, mendicant priests and lepers, and, periodically, the long retinue of a *daimyo* moving to or from Edo.

The society was rigidly structured in four classes (*Shi-no-ko-sho*), as prescribed by Confucian precepts. At the top was the *samurai* (loyal servant), a knight-administrator of the warrior class. He was to be unswervingly loyal, to the extreme of sacrificing his life, to his *daimyo*. The samurai were set apart from other members of the population by their privilege of wearing a long and a short sword. In an agrarian regime based on the cultivation of rice, the peasant ranked next to the samurai. Below him was the artisan; the bottom rank consisted of merchants. Their low status derived in part from the Confucian ethic that in an agricultural society, merchants were unproductive. Another contributing factor was the fear on the part of the shogunate that by accumulating wealth, the merchants might spawn revolt. Although this structure ensured the continuance of the Tokugawa regime, it also had shortcomings: it had the effect of stifling economic and social development in a sealed-off country.

At the beginning of the Tokugawa era, provisions for education were scant, and most of the samurai were illiterate. The period that followed showed a striking increase in literacy that pervaded all social classes but had its greatest impact with the samurai. Education was also based on Confucian philosophy, with its stress on moral training; "facts" were of secondary importance. A number of temple schools, *terakoya,* in the towns

---

[2]The terms Tokugawa, shogunate, and *Bakufu* will be used here interchangeably.

and the countryside served the peasants and the merchants; they were operated by Buddhist sects. The *Bakufu* set up schools for its retainers in Edo and in the *fudai* territories, which were under its direct administration. The *daimyo* established more than 200 clan schools for the samurai and their children. The principal college was the Shohei-ko in Edo, which taught the orthodox interpretation of Confucian doctrine.

As a result of these educational opportunities, the samurai emerged as a class of skillful administrators. They made possible an efficient government and formed an intellectual nucleus for the advance of scholarship.

Until the middle of the nineteenth century, medical training in the fief schools consisted of individual and group reading of Chinese texts, followed by group discussions. The students came from samurai families. So formal an atmosphere pervaded the medical classrooms that students would read the Chinese characters using a bizarre pronunciation, in order to set themselves apart. The teaching of materia medica was strongly emphasized and was based on the great Chinese herbal *Pen T'sao Kang Mu*.[3] A garden for the cultivation of medicinal plants was usually attached to a school. Dissection of the human body was forbidden, and anatomical charts were inaccurate, based as they were on theory and casual observation of the dismemberment of a beheaded corpse after an execution. Instruction in anatomy was restricted to the study of these charts. Examinations required the student to describe and explain selected passages from the Chinese classics, at times supplemented by practical questions on materia medica, diagnosis, and treatment.

Otherwise, most prospective practitioners of medicine gained their information as apprentices. They observed procedures, compounded medications, and read medical classics under guidance. They were sworn to secrecy about the special procedures they witnessed. A majority of the students were the sons of practitioners, since medicine was a hereditary profession.

The Portugese were the first Europeans to come to Japan, in about 1542-1543. In 1592, the Lusitanians were joined by Spaniards from the Philippines, since the Treaty of Tordesillas was no longer valid.[4] From their

---

[3]The *Pen T'sao* was compiled by Li Shih-chen by means of analyzing over 12,000 prescriptions. After twenty-seven years of unrelenting toil, he published the most effective medications as the *Pen T'sao*, late in the Ming period, circa A.D. 1596. In fifty-two volumes, it lists over 2,000 medications drawn from plant, animal, mineral, and other sources.

[4]In 1493, Pope Alexander VI (1431?-1503) issued a papal bull that fixed a line of demarcation for Portuguese and Spanish exploration of the world. It described a circle 100 leagues west of Cape Verde and through the poles. In 1494, Spain and Portugal signed a compact at Tordesillas, Spain, agreeing to the principle but moving the lines 370 leagues west. This placed all of the New World except Brazil in the Spanish realm. Japan was located in the half open to Portuguese trade and Christian missionary activity, while the Philippines lay in the Spanish sphere.

walled city, Manila, they had cast a covetous eye on Japan as a fertile field for conversion to Christianity.

The Portuguese made little effort to develop medicine in Japan. In part, their neglect owed to the fact that medicine was less advanced in the Iberian peninsula than in other European countries. Spain and Portugal were geographically isolated from the city states of northern Italy, where striking progress in medicine was being made. Scattered leprosaria, homes for foundlings, and a few small hospitals were the principal medical legacy of the Portuguese and the Spaniards.

The Japanese government accepted the Portuguese for several decades, but became increasingly suspicious that they might seize the country, as the Spaniards had conquered the Philippines. The tactics of the Portuguese Jesuits in due course antagonized the Japanese rulers; after the arrival of friars from Manila, open hostility broke out between the authorities and the Jesuits. Between 1614 and 1638, all Portuguese and Spaniards were expelled as Japan took the final steps for *sakoku*.

Nonetheless, the shogun, now Tokugawa Iemitsu (1604-1651), decided that he should maintain the existence of a slender thread to the Western world. For this purpose, the only recourse available to him was through the Dutch, who were operating a trading post at Hirado Island near the western tip of Kyushu.[5] The selection of the Dutch was buttressed by the consideration that they were non-Catholic and religion did not enter into their goals: they were solely concerned with trade and with overpowering their bitter rivals the Portuguese. For example, in 1637-1638, Dutch cannon supported Japanese armies in attacking Japanese Christian converts on the Shimabara peninsula; and the Dutch promptly tore down one of their warehouses on Hirado when a Japanese official complained that there was a Christian date on the cornerstone.

After the truce with Spain, the Dutch nation embarked on a remarkable ascent to world power. In the words of C. R. Boxer, the eminent maritime historian, "By 1648 the Dutch were indisputably the greatest trading nation in the world, with commercial outposts and fortified 'factories' scattered from Archangel to Recife and from New Amsterdam to Nagasaki. . . . This unprecedented achievement was mainly due to the dynamic energy and enterprise generated in the seaports of Holland and Zeeland."[6] As they had so far-flung an empire and so small a population, it was only natural that the Hollanders welcomed men from Germany, Sweden, Denmark, and Spain to serve in their fleets. Similarly, the doctors came from other countries, principally Germany. Since the United Provinces were in their "golden age," a medical career at home, which was bound to be lucrative, was for the medical men preferable to the dangers and limited opportunities that characterized the Dutch outposts and factories.

---

[5]The English had closed their short-lived factory at Hirado in 1623.

[6]Cr. R. Boxer, *The Dutch Seaborne Empire, 1600-1800* (New York: Alfred A. Knopf, 1965), p. 27.

The "golden age" of the Netherlands was reflected in the excellence of its medical schools, foremost among them Leyden. By the middle of the seventeenth century, the center of medical learning in Europe had moved across the Alps from the city states of northern Italy to the University of Leyden. The Netherlands did not apply religious discrimination to students from other countries, as did Roman Catholic France, and students from abroad, primarily England, were welcome to learn medicine at Leyden.

The faculty of medicine at Leyden reached its zenith under the brilliant Herman Boerhaave (1668-1738), who taught there from 1701 until his death. Boerhaave was a polymath who held simultaneous professorships in medicine, chemistry, and botany. He was described by Albrecht von Haller as *Communis Europae Praeceptor*—the teacher of all Europe. During the last decade of the eighteenth century, Vienna and Edinburgh began to replace Leyden as outstanding centers of medical education.

In the spring of 1641, the Tokugawa ordered the Dutch to move their factory from Hirado to Dejima in Nagasaki Bay. Dejima was an island stockade that had been built in 1634 by twenty-five prominent Nagasaki merchants, following the orders of the shogun, for guarding the handful of Portuguese traders allowed to remain in Japan. It was a small, fan-shaped island, 197 feet wide, and at its greatest length 706 feet. The security measures taken by the Japanese were so stringent that the Hollanders were literally imprisoned. The island was surrounded by a high wooden palisade, and the short bridge that connected it to the mainland was heavily guarded. Guards rowed around the sea walls both day and night, and the dozen Hollanders were spied upon by several hundred Japanese on the island. The staff of the Dutch trading post included an *opperhoofd* (captain), clerks, and almost always a doctor, who might be a Swede or a German as well as a Hollander. For these men, the only real opportunity to see the land of their captors came with the colorful annual *hofreis* to Edo, a trip made for the purpose of reporting to the shogun on the state of all countries where they traded and on the activities of the hated Portuguese. They were also expected to present gifts. Save for the *hofreis*, when they were still guarded by a large Japanese retinue, the Hollanders were allowed only an occasional visit to Nagasaki, to enjoy the charms of the geisha. For each such expedition, a special writ from the Nagasaki *Bugyo* (shogun's magistrate or minister) had to be obtained. The Dutch sustained themselves by their annual trade with Batavia, basing their commerce on one or more East Indiamen that sailed from Batavia to Nagasaki at the time of the summer monsoon.

At first, three seemingly insurmountable barriers obstructed the exchange of information between the Japanese and the Dutch: the formidable language problem, owing to the great difficulty the Japanese had in mastering a European language; the harsh restrictions on contacts; and the ban on Western books. This last, the ban, had been issued by Tokugawa Iemitsu in 1630 when he forbade the importation of thirty-two Western books on scientific and religious topics that had been translated into Chinese by the great Jesuit missionary in Peking, Matteo Ricci (1552-1610). This ban severed the Japanese from all sources of Western knowledge except the Dutch. Yet there were always some Japanese who were undaunted in their pursuit of Western learning, mainly medicine, and they regarded Dejima as their classroom. Because of the tight controls there, some disguised themselves as menials in order to gain entry.

Only the *Oranda tsuji* ("Holland interpreters") were allowed access to the foreigners. Their positions were hereditary, and they ranked as governmental representatives. A mutual lack of trust prevailed because of the lingering affection of the *Oranda tsuji* for the Portuguese, whose language they continued to use until the end of the seventeenth century. Yet they sought knowledge about Western medical practice from the Dejima doctors, and in turn they were willing to violate official decrees by giving the doctors information on the culture, natural history, and medicine of Japan.

For more than a millennium the Japanese followed a system of medicine that they called *Kampo* (Han technique). They had adopted it from China during the tremendous cultural appropriation that occurred in the seventh century, at the height of the T'ang dynasty (A.D. 618-906).

Medicines were drawn from the massive Chinese materia medica and from native products: the two most widely used were ginseng and antler. Medications often contained as many as a dozen ingredients, and there was little specificity in therapeusis. The most popular procedure was acupuncture, in which slender, solid needles were inserted into specified points in the skin. The points were believed to lead to an extensive network of ducts that in turn fed into twelve major channels—six for *yin* and six for *yang*.[7] Each channel related to a major organ, and disease was treated by the insertion of needles into points along meridians that represented the diseased organ. A variation on this procedure was moxibustion, in which burning cones of mugwort, *mogusa,* were applied to the acupuncture points. While acupuncture was the more popular treatment with the Chinese, the Japanese preferred moxibustion.

During the two centuries that passed between the sealing off of Japan by its government, so fearful of contact with the West in the mid-seventeenth century, and the "opening" of the nation in the middle of the nineteenth century, European medical knowledge nevertheless managed to penetrate the "closed" country. The eventual triumph of Western medicine represented a victory both for those Japanese students who sought knowledge of the West, and also for a small number of notable European physicians who served over the years as the resident doctor at Dejima. These men were, in chronological sequence of their service, Willem Ten

[7]Two opposing forces, *yang,* masculine, and *yin,* feminine, were supposed to be omnipresent, including the human body in their influence. It was thought that if the "harmony" between the individual and his environment or within the body was lost, disease would result.

Rhijne, Engelbert Kaempfer, Carl Pieter Thunberg, and Philipp von Siebold.

The prisonlike conditions at Dejima, with their concomitant lack of opportunities for the practice of medicine, were not an attractive prospect to most physicians. Despite these obstacles, Ten Rhijne and the others were eager to study an exotic, romantic land and did come there, where they taught medicine and natural history to the Japanese. Their students in turn told these doctors about a Japan that was unknown to the West.

The Nagasaki interpreters were the first students to learn Western medicine, and they passed on their information to other Japanese. Less than one decade after the gates at Dejima were closed on the Dutch, four Japanese youths asked Caspar Schamberger, a German barber-surgeon, to teach them his methods of wound treatment. When he came to Edo on the *hofreis* in 1650, the Western doctor's instruction attracted so many Japanese that henceforth the Dejima doctor was always made a member of the mission. Schamberger's techniques were described in what may have been the first treatise on Western therapeutics, *Komo-geka* ("surgery of the red hairs").[8] In 1665 the first certificate of a degree of competency in Western medicine was issued at Dejima to Arashiyama Choan, stating that he was "well instructed in the art of surgery. He is therefore well acquainted with the potency of Dutch medicines . . . and we hereby declare him to be an accomplished practitioner."[9]

The facility of the interpreters in the Dutch language was expanded in 1671, when the shogun ordered the *opperhoofd* to instruct them in reading and writing Dutch. This directive signaled another recognition on the part of the Japanese government of the importance of communicating with the West.

In 1674-76, Willem Ten Rhijne (1647-1700), a graduate of the celebrated Faculty of Medicine at Leyden, became the first scholar-physician to serve at Dejima. His chief interest lay in studying and documenting the medical practices of *Kampo*. From his observations emerged the first comprehensive description of acupuncture: *Dissertatio de arthritide. . .* (1683).

A monumental and unprecedented cultural breakthrough to the West, in the form of a detailed account of the history, culture, and medical practices of Japan, *The History of Japan. . .* (1727), was the work of the remarkable German physician Engelbert Kaempfer (1651-1716). Shortly after he arrived in Dejima in 1690, Kaempfer began to teach a young Japanese "appointed to wait upon me as my servant and at the same time to be instructed by me in physick and surgery."[10] Medical practitioners of the court evinced their curiosity about Western medicine by asking Kaempfer innumerable questions when he came to Edo on the *hofreis*. Their queries covered such a variety of topics as the severity of diseases,

---

[8]It should be noted that *komo* carries a pejorative force.

[9]C. R. Boxer, *Jan Compagnie in Japan,* 1600-1850 (The Hague: Martinus Nijhoff, 1950), p. 46.

[10]Engelbert Kaempfer, *The History of Japan,* trans. J. S. Scheuchzer (London, 1727), I, ii.

the treatment of internal disorders, and the physician's ultimate goal—a drug to bestow immortality.

Japanese interest in Western medicine continued to grow. A work entitled *Geka Soden* ("surgery handed down"), the first extensive Japanese compilation on European surgery, was published in 1706 by Narabayashi Chinzan (1648-1711), a Nagasaki interpreter.

Another advance for Japanese students of Western learning was made in 1720 with the assistance of the progressive Shogun Tokugawa Yoshimune (1678-1751). He was advised that the Japanese calendar, the nation's almanac, was inaccurate but that it could not be corrected without recourse to hitherto banned Chinese texts, these in turn consisting of translations of Western texts on astronomy and mathematics. Yoshimune directed that the ban be lifted. He gave further stimulus to the study of the Dutch language when, in 1740, he ordered a court physician, Noro Genjo, to learn Western medicine and Aoki Konyo (1698-1769), the court librarian, to compile a Dutch dictionary. Published in 1758, Aoki's word book, although incomplete, was a minor landmark in the advance of Western learning.

A major landmark, indeed the most important achievement in the dissemination of Western medicine, was the translation of a European anatomy text. This feat was accomplished in 1774 by Sugita Gempaku (1733-1817) and Maeno Ryotaku (1723-1791) when they published *Kaitai Shinsho,* based on the translation of a Dutch version of the German Johann Adam Kulmus's *Anatomische Tabellen (Tabulae anatomicae in quibus corporis humani,* Danzig, 1722). The two Japanese scholars had obtained copies of Kulmus's work and wished to compare his illustrations with the distribution of organs in a Japanese corpse. When they were allowed to observe the dismemberment of a beheaded criminal in 1771, Sugita and Maeno were struck by the fact that what they saw was contrary to what appeared in native anatomical charts. Thus, with only a fragmentary knowledge of Dutch, they determined to undertake the enormous task of translating Kulmus's work, a project that took three arduous years. Illustrated with wood-block prints, their book further advanced the cause of Western medicine: Japanese who were unable to read Dutch texts could now study an accurate description of human anatomy. As the first European text to be translated by Japanese and printed and published in Japan, *Kaitai Shinsho* was truly a milestone.

The publication of *Kaitai Shinsho* opened an era of more intensive Western study, concentrated most heavily on medicine, natural history, and the Dutch language. This period is known as *Rangaku* ("Dutch study"): Dutch versions of German texts in anatomy, pharmacology, internal medicine, and surgery were translated into Japanese by *Rangakusha* (Dutch scholars). Twelve private schools offering instruction in Western medicine and Dutch were established in Edo, Miyako, and Osaka. Otsuki Gentaku (1757-1827), the leading *Rangakusha* in Edo, opened Shirando Juku in

1786, where more than ninety students enrolled. His was the dominant voice in proclaiming the superiority of European science over Chinese.

In 1823, when the enthusiasm for *Rangaku* was at its height, the most memorable physician of the *sakoku* period arrived at Dejima. Philipp Franz Balthasar von Siebold (1796-1866), a German, was the first to teach the Japanese the diagnosis and treatment of disease as practiced in the West. At the same time, he amassed a huge and diverse personal collection of things Japanese.

A painstaking teacher, Siebold attracted so many students that he became the first foreigner to give organized instruction on the mainland. After practicing physicians joined the student body, larger quarters became essential, and Siebold was granted a home in Narutaki, on a Nagasaki hillside. As his fame spread, many practitioners from Nagasaki and more distant communities referred patients to him, often accompanying them in order to attend his classes. It was, ironically, Siebold's zeal for what amounted to hoarding Japanese treasures that precipitated his imprisonment on Dejima and subsequent expulsion. His treasonous act was to obtain through bribery a copy of the secret map that would reveal Japan's geographical vulnerabilities to an invader.

Siebold's greatest legacy to Japan was his former students. They founded medical schools and translated and wrote medical texts, thereby giving further impetus to the advance of Western medicine. One of them, Ito Genboku, opened Shosendo Juku in Edo in 1833, and two years later, Ko Ryosai, the first Japanese to practice ophthalmology, opened Chozendo Juku in Osaka. Ito's understanding of the importance of practical training with European physicians prompted him to persuade the *Bakufu* in 1861 to sponsor two of his best students, Ito Gempaku and Hayashi Kenkai, for the study of medicine in the Netherlands.

Another of Ito's pupils and the last of the great *Rangaku* doctors was Ogata Koan, who opened Tekitekisai Juku in Osaka in 1838. Ogata is revered in Japan today as the man who embodied the finest qualities of the teacher and the physician. The devotion that he inspired in his students was expressed in the writings of Fukuzawa Yukichi (1835-1901), who became a highly effective advocate of the liberal political concepts and standards of the West: in 1858 he founded *Keiogijuku*, which developed into one of Japan's leading private universities. Nagayo Sensai, another pupil of Ogata, wrote the first public-health code in Japan.

Thus, by the middle of the nineteenth century, Western medicine had gained a firm foothold in Japan. A core of enlightened physicians understood its supremacy over *Kampo* and were eager to propagate its benefits. The ban on Western contacts had been eased and an increasing (albeit still small) number of physicians could communicate in Dutch. It was at this time that Otto Mohnike, another German came to Dejima.

2

Otto Mohnike

Otto Gottlieb Johann Mohnike (1814-1887), a German physician, introduced vaccination and the stethoscope and wrote a thorough account of the state of Japanese health in the middle of the nineteenth century. Despite these contributions, he has received little attention in Japanese medical history.

The son of Gottlieb Christian Frederick Mohnike and his wife, Eleonora Carolina Ulrica von Sticker, Otto Mohnike was born in Stralsund on June 27, 1814. He matriculated as a student on November 4, 1833, at the Faculty of Medicine at the Royal Prussian Rhineland University of Bonn, the newest of the German universities. The perceptiveness of Mohnike's studies is attributable to his excellent educational background, which bore the stamp of the emphasis on medical science that characterized the German medical schools in his student days. After graduating, he determined to see the wider world and followed the trail of other German medical explorers to the Netherlands. There he received a commission as a medical officer, third class, in the Military Medical Corps of the East Indies and sailed for Batavia on July 28, 1844, arriving there four months later.[1]

In Java, Mohnike encountered the disease problems of a tropical country with a large, illiterate indigenous population that relied primarily on native practitioners. It suffered recurrent epidemics of cholera, with a high mortality; thousands of natives, as well as a number of Europeans, died from other enteric fevers each year. Malaria was prevalent and uncontrolled. Although the incidence of leprosy was declining, as in other lands, programs and facilities for isolating lepers were almost nonexistent. When the first Dutch founded the fort of Batavia next to the native capital, Djakarta, in 1619, beriberi was widespread and believed to be caused by an exotic infectious agent. In the middle of the nineteenth century this theory was still accepted.[2]

The native population lived under wretched socioeconomic conditions: inadequate shelter, an absence of sanitation, and gross malnutrition; all these exacerbated the disease problem. The availability of preventive and

[1] Archives of the Ministry of Colonies, No. 2704, p. 254, at Algemeen Rijksarchief, The Hague. This and other information on Mohnike, courtesy of Mrs. M.C.J.C. Jansen van Hoff, Archivist of the First Section.

[2] D. Schoute, *De Geneeskunde in den Dienst der Oost-Indische Compagnie in Nederlandsch-Indie* (Amsterdam: J. H. DeBussey, 1929), p. 126.

curative services was severely limited by the geographical inaccessibility of the people, who were unconcerned about their state of health.

The only trained native practitioners were a small number of *doktors-djawa* who had been taught the technique of vaccination at the military hospital in Weltvreden, the Dutch community at Batavia.[3] Apart from the handful of *doktors-djawa,* the natives relied on untrained indigenous practitioners and midwives.

Newly arrived and lower-ranking medical officers such as Mohnike were posted to outlying stations, where the duties were demanding, the health hazards great, and the disease problems nearly overwhelming. For his work during a typhoid epidemic in 1846-47, Mohnike was awarded a knighthood in the Order of the Netherlands Lion. In November 1847, he was promoted and assigned to duty at Dejima, where he arrived in August 1848. It was a propitious time for a foreign scholar. He was allowed to immerse himself in the medical problems of Japan to a greater degree than his predecessors could, his movements were less restricted, and the climate among Japanese practitioners was hospitable. The latter were applying Western methods in a number of fiefs, with the approval of their *daimyo.* The physicians to the *Bakufu* openly pursued Western medicine. The *opperhoofd* at Dejima, Joseph Henrij Levijssohn, gave his full support to Mohnike's scholarly pursuits.

At Dejima, Mohnike compiled his reports on medical practices on the basis of his contacts with patients, discussions with Japanese physicians, and his observations of Japanese life. For detailed information on Kampo, he referred to a translation into Dutch of *Sotokeikenzensho* ("complete study of all tumors").

In Chinese-Japanese traditional medicine (*Kampo*), the "magic number" was five. It was held that five factors contributed to disease: wind, air, heat, cold, and weakness. These in turn related to five elements, five plants, five basic colors, and five "viscera": heart, liver, lungs, kidney, and spleen. Thus there existed a total of twenty-five major categories of disease with numerous subdivisions. Disease resulted from the movement of a basic factor from one organ to another.

Mohnike described the detailed diagnostic procedure of palpation of the pulse.[4] The frequency of irregularities of the pulse was used to predict

[3] It soon became apparent that the *doktors-djawa* were called on to treat a wide range of medical problems, and in 1864 the course was lengthened to three years. In 1875 it was divided into a two-year premedical and a three-year medical program; the premedical course was extended to three years in 1881. The school was significantly strengthened in 1888, when it was merged with the pathology and bacteriology laboratories of the military hospital. Two years later, the language of instruction became Dutch. A. de Waart, M.D., "Medical education in the Dutch East Indies," in *Addresses and Papers, Dedication Ceremonies and Medical Conference, Peking Union Medical College* (Peking, 1922).

[4] "They have a twofold way of examining the pulse. . . . They examine the *arteria radialis* either in five different places or at a single one using three fingers of the hand. They always feel the pulse at both wrists and pay meticulous attention to any real or imaginary deviation

the length of time that the patient would survive. If the pulse skipped every third beat, it was supposed that the patient would die on the third day; if every other beat, on the following day. All in all, practitioners distinguished twenty-four different categories of the pulse.

Medical training continued to be on the apprenticeship system, and a candidate often studied under several preceptors. The most popular medical men in Edo and Miyako might have as many as fifty apprentices, and each of them paid a high fee. There were no controls over the practice of medicine and no examinations to determine the candidate's competency.

According to Mohnike, in the middle of the nineteenth century, the only institution in Japan ranked by the natives as a university was Seido, founded by the Tokugawa shogunate at Edo in 1690. Mohnike, however, termed it

not a university in the European sense of the word but an academy for scholars occupied exclusively with the higher study of the Chinese language and literature and the explanation of religious and philosophical writings, principally those of Confucius. The inscription over the entrance to the school, translated, reads: "entrance to the most precious treasures."[5]

Medical practitioners were divided into several categories. The largest group were general practitioners who treated a wide range of disorders; those who worked in rural areas were, in Mohnike's judgment, no better than the untrained native practitioners, the *dokoens,* in the Netherlands East Indies. Practitioners who specialized in surgery, internal medicine, ophthalmology, diseases of the mouth, obstetrics, and fractures and dislocations settled in the larger cities. There were also practitioners of acupuncture and moxibustion, masseurs, and midwives. Since Japanese medical men compounded their own prescriptions, pharmacies on the European pattern did not exist. Instead, small shops scattered in the rural areas sold simple medicines.

An ambivalent attitude about medicine had become apparent in the empire. The shogunate employed a total of forty-five practitioners, who were presumably restricted to applying Chinese medicine but who furtively used Western techniques; and a number of the outer *daimyo* relied exclusively on Western medicine. The large number of physicians employed by the shogunate and *daimyo* was, in Mohnike's view, "more for ostentation than out of necessity."[6]

---

from normal. They alternate between pressing their fingers gently and firmly. When they apply three fingers to the right wrist at the same time they believe that the first finger will elicit [awareness of] any disease of the lung or large intestine; the second finger . . . disorders of the spleen or stomach; and the third, disorders in the San-sho and Meimong." Otto Mohnike, "Aanteekeningen over de Geneeskunde der Japanezen," *Het Geneeskundig Tijdschrift voor Nederlansch-Indië,* 1853, *1:* 283-84.

[5]Ibid., p. 220.

[6]Ibid., p. 217.

Practitioners with no court affiliations ranked with civil servants and artisans. They were permitted to wear a special garment, a *hakama* (a trouserlike pleated skirt), and to carry a single sword. On the other hand, personal physicians to the shogunate and the major *daimyo* were attired like high military officers and nobility and were permitted to carry two swords, if that dignity had been awarded to their masters. When actively practicing their calling, they found the wearing of a surrogate bamboo sword more convenient.

Physicians could also be differentiated by their hairstyle: those in the service of the shogun and the high-ranking *daimyo* shaved their heads, as did Buddhist monks. Other doctors braided their hair in a special way.

Mohnike described the knowledge of Western medicine as "limited, disconnected, superficial, and aphoristic," yet he admired the Japanese determination to learn it despite great difficulties.[7] A lack of suitable dictionaries was a major impediment. The sole resource was the Dutch-Japanese lexicon that had been compiled by Hendrik Doeff (1777-1835), the *opperhoofd* at Dejima from 1803 to 1817.[8] A Japanese-Dutch dictionary, compiled by Philipp von Siebold, was available only in manuscript form.

The lack of programs in hygiene and sanitation shocked Mohnike, since in other respects Japan followed a more enlightened policy toward the welfare of her citizens than did any other non-European country. Yet he saw a bright future if only *sakoku* were to be abolished:

> If ever . . . the country comes under the rule of a monarch with the will and power to give a European civilization to the Japanese nation . . . as Peter the Great has done for the Russians, then . . . the Japanese will make speedier and greater progress in the different branches of medicine than in the other arts and sciences.[9]

Moxibustion, the most popular Japanese therapeutic procedure, was used by practically every citizen for almost every disorder. The usual technique was to place two rows of moxa, each containing seven balls, on the skin at a site selected for its supposed relationship to the disorder. The procedure was repeated daily or every third day for two or three weeks. Many healthy persons used moxibustion as a springtime prophylactic against summer fevers, "just as in Europe many still are accustomed to having a blood-letting done in the Spring."[10]

[7]Ibid., p. 246.

[8]Known as *Nagasaki Halma* or *Doyaku Halma*, it had been completed in 1833 by Doeff's Japanese colleagues but was not published until 1855-1858; it was based largely on the Dutch-French dictionary *Nieuw Nederduitsch en Fransch Woordenboek* (Amsterdam, 1717), by François Halma (1655-1722). Doeff's dictionary and that of Fujibayashi Fuzan, *Yaku-ken*, published in 1810, were both based on an enormous lexicon, *Haruma wage* (also *Edo wage*), of which only thirty copies had been published, in 1796.

[9]Mohnike, "Aanteekeningen over de Geneeskunde der Japanezen," pp. 43-44.

[10]Ibid., p. 293.

The moxa was a woolly substance found in the leaves of one of the half-dozen varieties of *Artemesia*. If the leaves were older and had been dried for an extended period, the moxa was supposed to have greater curative powers.

The Japanese traced the introduction of the moxa and acupuncture to the sixth century, when both were imported from China. Moxibustion was popular throughout Central Asia and as far west as the river Don in Russia, but it had not been adopted in Europe until the publication of Engelbert Kaempfer's *The History of Japan,* in 1727.

According to Mohnike, moxa was applied to the area between the nose and mouth for the treatment of a stroke, for lethargy, and for psychological disorders. For jaundice, the balls were placed over the right and left hypochondrium. In the treatment of an abscess or bubo, one large cone was applied on the swelling to hasten maturation and to allow drainings of the pus through the eschar; by this means the practitioner was spared from using a lance, which, because it penetrated the human body, he would avoid at all cost.

Since moxibustion provided such a popular, effective, and almost painless remedy, Mohnike questioned why it was not used in Europe in place of harsher caustics:

The European burning cylinders, often an inch long, made from elder pith or cotton and moistened with ether or turpentine, are used by our surgeons only in extreme cases because of the unbearable pain they produce. Although these are also called *moxas* they are not to be compared with the Japanese cones, which are applied even to women and children without causing them to flinch.[11]

Acupuncture was almost as popular with the Japanese as moxibustion. Mohnike tested it by inserting needles into the hearts and lungs of dogs and noted no discernible results. He concluded that it had "only very little therapeutic effect, or even none at all."[12] In all instances thin needles were favored, since they were believed to have a "strengthening" effect; thick needles, which at times drew a drop of blood, were considered to have a weakening effect.

As with moxibustion, the people felt no hesitation at inserting the needles into each other or even into themselves. They might also call in strolling acupuncturists, who were usually blind, and who advertised with special bells the excellence of their art, as they walked with other peddlers along the lanes at dusk.

The Japanese sought with equal frequency the services of a masseur (*anma*) who were also usually blind, for rheumatic pains in the arms, shoulders, or back, and for fatigue after a tiring journey. The technique

---

[11]Ibid., pp. 293-94.
[12]Ibid., p. 298.

consisted of pressing, tapping, and massaging specific points according to the location of the pain. Frequently the manipulation was supplemented by the use of a wooden instrument consisting of a crosspiece with small wheels at the ends, which was rolled over the skin with varying degrees of pressure.

Mohnike deplored Japanese therapeutics as "highly irrational, symptomatic, and ineffectual."[13] Before the arrival of the Portuguese in 1542-43, the Japanese had slavishly followed the enormous Chinese formulary. The Lusitanians introduced several hitherto unknown medications such as Egyptian mummy, saffron, and the tusk of the narwhal, *Monodon monoceros,* all of which gained instant popularity among Japanese practitioners. After the closure of the empire, Western medications continued to be popular, and the Dutch imported them from Europe and from their trading posts in Africa and Asia. During Mohnike's three years at Nagasaki, the purchase of medicines still represented a small but highly lucrative share of the annual trade, which was controlled by the *Bakufu.*

Mohnike compiled an extensive catalog of therapeutic agents from mineral, animal, and vegetable sources used by practitioners of traditional medicine. The principal medicines of mineral origin were cinnabar for syphilis, sodium and magnesium sulfates as antiphlogistic agents and purgatives, potassium nitrate as an antiphlogistic and diuretic, slaked lime as an antacid and for the control of external bleeding, a mixture of alum and mercury for advanced syphilis, antimony sulfide for skin disease and scrofula, and ferric sulfate for internal and external bleeding. An unusual therapeutic agent was prepared by leaving a stalk of bamboo packed with table salt in a public urinal for several days. When the stalk and its contents were thoroughly saturated with urine, the salt was applied to noma or other ulcerations of the oral cavity.

Animal products enjoyed more popularity than did mineral derivatives. Powdered narwhal tusk or rhinoceros horn was used for diseases of the chest, as an emollient, and to control hematemesis. A decoction from tusk was considered efficacious in the treatment of smallpox. The Japanese favored the popular Oriental practice of applying cups carved from rhinoceros horn to the skin for their special power to locate and neutralize any poisonous substance in the human body. The bile of a bear was used externally as a salve and internally to stimulate digestion and to eradicate intestinal worms. Ambergris and musk were used for abdominal cramps. The nests of the bird *Cypselus esculentus,* imported from the East Indies, were prepared as a decoction and administered as a nutrient and to stimulate the manufacture of blood.

Extracts from the reptiles *Trigonocephalus Blomhoffi* and *Hydrophis colubrina* were applied in powdered form for skin diseases, including

---

[13]Ibid., p. 284.

syphilis and leprosy, and were also taken internally for paralytic states. Disorders of the urinary tract, including hematuria, calculus, and urinary retention, were treated with extracts from the lizards *Scincus quinque-lineatus* and the common Chinese gekko, *Platydaetylus Guttatus.* A pulverized preparation from the toad *Bufo Vulgaris* was believed to cure scabies, chronic ulcers, and other skin diseases; in the form of a decoction, it was recommended for a variety of intestinal disorders as well as for epilepsy and cramps. Mohnike noted that powdered toad had also been used in his native Germany as a remedy against *Tinea Capitis:* "The heads of children suffering from this disease are covered with a thick layer of carbonized, pulverized toads."[14]

Pearls from Kyushu were pulverized and applied externally for diseases of the eye and ear; they were taken internally for gastrointestinal disorders. The only remedies popular in China but shunned by the Japanese were those prepared from the excreta of animals.

Japanese practitioners drew on such vegetable sources as aloe wood to strengthen the nerves and the stomach, and sandalwood to arrest bleeding. Benzoin served as an expectorant, and asafoedita as an antispasmodic and antihelminthic.

Lithotomy and herniotomy were unknown, and, although hydrocele and cysts were common, no surgical procedures were undertaken for their removal. Even the extraction of a tooth was viewed with alarm. During two centuries of peace, Japanese practitioners had no opportunity to practice surgical skills on battle casualties. Contrasting this with the European experience of military conflict as a stimulus to the advancement of surgery, Mohnike suggested:

For the sake of surgery in Japan, it might be desirable if the country were drawn into a war, for then many doctors would have the chance and even the necessity of bringing into practice what they now know only from European books, and thus improve themselves by the experience.[15]

Mohnike opined that the small number of Japanese doctors who had begun to undertake surgical procedures were more dexterous and meticulous in ligating blood vessels than were European surgeons. Yet the techniques they practiced and most of the instruments they used had long since been discarded in Europe.

On the other hand, the Japanese manufactured surgical instruments of high quality that were modeled after European products. With technological training, Mohnike concluded, they would be able to match those of Europe. He acquired a set of lancets made in Nagasaki that he considered equal to the best obtainable in Paris. He also preferred the Japanese paper

[14]Ibid., p. 335.
[15]Ibid., p. 286.

dressings to the linen ones used in Europe: "I have discovered . . . that some kinds of . . . Japanese paper dressings . . . are excellent for surgical cases and even preferable to the new English machine-made pads."[16]

Mohnike had the highest praise for Japanese dentures:

They have great experience in inserting both single teeth and whole dentures, using either natural, human teeth, or imitations of ivory, narwhal tusk, or porcelain. I do not think that the Japanese can be surpassed in this field by European dentists. People I talked with almost daily for a year seemed to have all of their teeth. Later I learned to my great surprise that they did not have a single one of their own teeth. In fact, Japanese dentures are to be preferred over those made in Europe, because they are more hygienic and durable.[17]

In the larger cities, maternity care combined European techniques with native ones. Mohnike praised the originality of Japanese prints illustrating obstetrical texts: they contrasted sharply with the reproductions of European drawings that accompanied native texts in other fields.

He found some of the obstetrical procedures fearsome: "In difficult births, obstetrical intervention usually consists of pulling the child out by senseless, traumatic, and almost brutal procedures."[18] Mohnike cited one gruesome technique that was resorted to when the fetus could not be extracted with forceps. An instrument resembling a windlass with a large loop at the end of its cable was inserted in the vagina: "In very difficult cases . . . hook and cable are attached to the child and an attempt is made to wind it out of the uterus and the pelvic cavity as if one were weighing an anchor from the bottom of the sea. It is needless to note that the fetus is always destroyed by such violent surgery and often the mother as well."[19]

Obstetrical forceps were made of whalebone instead of metal; one model had closed blades similar to the instrument developed by Jean Palfyn (1649-1730) in Paris more than a century earlier. There were also hooks, levers, and staves with a noose at the end for grasping the fetal head.

Caesarean section and decapitation were unknown. Internal version was carried out with singular skill because of the manual dexterity and small hands of the Japanese. Maternal and infant mortality after normal delivery were rare; maternal morbidity, when it occurred, was attributable to two harmful native procedures. One required the prospective mother to wear a cloth several inches wide, *Iwata-obi* (a sash worn tightly around the abdomen).[20] It was applied at the time of the first fetal movements and was

---

[16]Ibid., p. 288.
[17]Ibid., p. 300.
[18]Ibid., p. 326.
[19]Ibid., p. 336.
[20]The application of the *Iwata-obi* was cause for a family celebration. When the wife of one of the shogun's retainers became pregnant, he sent an official *obi*, which became a family treasure.

worn until two or three months after delivery. The custom had originated in the belief that otherwise the fetus would become too large and would be deformed. The second practice was to place the mother, immediately after delivery, in a kneeling position for nine days and nights with only a small prop under each elbow as her supports. Prolapse of the uterus and profuse postpartum hemorrhage frequently resulted.

The prevalence of eye disease and blindness was staggering: "In ophthalmology the Japanese are still far behind the West; as a proof of this one has only to observe the multitude of blind people in the country, some of whom have lost their vision because of smallpox, another group theirs because of other, poorly treated eye infections."[21] Mohnike suggested that the high incidence of eye diseases might be attributed to the Japanese hairstyle, which left the head uncovered. Chronic and poorly treated diseases of the eye constituted a large part of Mohnike's practice; he was told that in Edo, with a population estimated at five million, there were 50,000 blind persons. He reckoned that seven out of ten patients with a simple catarrhal inflammation of the eye were destined to suffer permanent diminution of vision. The major cause was the use of harsh medications, which provoked severe irritation. The ancient technique of "couching," in which a needle was inserted through the cornea to dislocate the opaque lens, was the only operative procedure for cataract. Although there were a few fairly skillful eye doctors in Edo and Miyako, Mohnike unhappily concluded that ophthalmology in Japan was practiced at the same low level as in Java.

Leprosy existed in all parts of the empire, from the most tropical areas in southern Kyushu to the frigid regions of northern Hokkaido, but there were no regulations whatsoever to control the spread of the disease. Lepers were not isolated but continued in their daily occupations, eating and sleeping with their families in crowded, nonventilated homes. Since there were no leprosaria, patients with advanced disease occasionally endeavored to isolate themselves at home, a highly unsatisfactory gesture.

A Japanese physician estimated that the proportion of lepers was one in ten thousand inhabitants; thus, with a population estimated at about thirty-five million, the country had 3,500 lepers. This represented a lower incidence than that in Java and Sumatra.

Although Mohnike treated high-ranking persons who were suffering from the early stages of leprosy, it remained essentially a disease of the poor; then he made the *hofreis,* he was besieged by lepers begging alms along the Tokaido. He had never seen patients so terribly disfigured, and their way of life was wretched:

They are forced into this nomadic existence by the poverty of their relatives, who are unable to care for them, and by their own inability to earn a living. Some of

[21]Mohnike, "Aanteekeningen over de Geneeskunde der Japanezen," p. 288.

them live in pits that they have dug in the dirt along the roadside like the lairs of wild animals. They crawled naked from their pits when they heard us approach and begged the stranger for alms. Never in my life have I seen such pitiful and grotesque faces.[22]

Scabies was common among all classes, in both sexes and at all ages. The greatest number of cases occurred in the spring, and the large blisters frequently became chronic indolent ulcers. The scabies mite, larger than the European one, was easily visible to the naked eye, and Mohnike frequently observed sufferers who were digging the mite out of the side of a sore.

Syphilis, which could be traced to the arrival of the Portuguese in the middle of the sixteenth century, was now widespread. In contrast to the West, where the infection was kept hidden, "Nobody makes a secret of being afflicted by syphilis and no more or less importance is attached to it than to any mild physical disorder."[23] Although the disease was common and treatment inadequate, tertiary syphilis was rare. Mohnike saw no more than three or four persons who had lost their noses from it and observed only a single case of syphilitic necrosis of the frontal bone. He concluded that, as in most European countries, syphilis had become more virulent since the sixteenth century. Climatic conditions he considered to be a major determinant of its virulence; these, he thought, accounted for the fact that in Japan, with its cyclical climate, the disease was less severe than in tropical Java.

Mohnike had high praise for the control of prostitution:

In perhaps no other country in the world is public prostitution officially regulated and meticulously supervised as in Japan. . . . It is an integral part of the present-day machinery of state. At the same time it has the most intimate connection with the entire social life of the nation.[24]

The number of brothels seemed out of proportion to the population when compared with the situation in Europe: no town of any size was without at least one. For example, at a new village just four years old on a small island in the Inland Sea, with 321 inhabitants residing in 49 houses, there was a brothel housing twenty-seven prostitutes. In Nagasaki, with a population of no more than 33,000 people, two lanes were lined with twenty-four brothels, in which a total of 650 prostitutes worked. Similarly, Mohnike found the Tokaido "with the exception of some mountainous areas, almost literally one uninterrupted chain of hotels, resting places, inns, and brothels."[25] In Mohnike's opinion, the popularity of prostitution

[22]Ibid., p. 224.
[23]Ibid., p. 229.
[24]Ibid., p. 230.
[25]Ibid., p. 231.

could be attributed to the Japanese enjoyment of sexuality, which appeared to exceed that of all other nations.[26]

Most of the prostitutes came from poor rural families and had been sold at or before puberty to a brothel keeper at a price fixed by the government in accordance with the grade of the brothel. Police regulations directed that these new girls could not practice the trade until they were fifteen years old, but this was often ignored: "Since their physical development is accelerated in these hotbeds of sin, we may safely assume that most of the girls are initiated in all secrets of Venus *vulgivaga* long before they are fifteen."[27]

The terms of their sale stipulated that the girls serve in the brothel until the age of twenty-five, after which they could return to their families, not infrequently to become the wives of respected citizens. Prostitution was not regarded as a repugnant profession, and women of status and rank often enjoyed the friendship of a prostitute without sullying their own reputations. Patrons of the most famous prostitutes also suffered no demeaning of repute.

The social acceptance of the prostitute was ascribed in part to a historical event. During a civil war in A.D. 1185, the mikado was overthrown, he died, and his impoverished concubines had no alternative to becoming prostitutes on the streets of Miyako. His subjects concluded that if women who had enjoyed the most intimate physical relations with the mikado offered their bodies to the public, prostitution could not be degrading.

A second reason for the acceptance of prostitution arose from the Confucian ethic of parental devotion. A girl who had been sold to a brothel traditionally supported her parents by her earnings, thus sacrificing herself for their benefit. On the other hand, owners of brothels, according to Mohnike, were relegated to the ignominious caste of the *eta*, the executioners and cattle slaughterers.[28]

Each street in a brothel district was assigned to a police warden, whose responsibility it was to see that the prostitutes were well fed and clothed and were not abused by either their customers or the owners of the house. Furthermore, although there were no routine medical inspections of prostitutes for venereal disease as there were in Europe, the law required brothel owners to retain the services of one or more medical practitioners to ensure that if a prostitute contracted a venereal disease she would receive prompt treatment. As a further measure against the spread of venereal disease, prostitutes were not allowed to engage in their profession anywhere other than in a regulated brothel, or in a teahouse.

[26]This would seem a questionable observation, considering that cramped living quarters must have drastically reduced the rate of intercourse at home.

[27]Mohnike, "Aanteekeningen over de Geneeskunde der Japanezen," pp. 252-3.

[28]This observation would certainly not apply to the owners of the famous geisha houses in Kyoto and Edo.

The police used the brothels as observation posts for surveillance of the citizens and the apprehension of outlaws:

. . . for observing the people in their most secret and unguarded hours of pleasure. To this end every visitor has to sign his name and address in a book when he enters the brothel. The owner of the house is under strict legal obligation to notify the police immediately if a suspect is using his premises. Most criminals, especially thieves and swindlers, are discovered and caught in brothels, very often by the prostitutes themselves.[29]

The strict governmental regulation of opium use stood in sharp contrast to the uncontrolled trade in other strong medicinals and poisons. The sale of opium by a practitioner was strictly forbidden without a written permit from the local authority and the endorsement of two responsible persons who guaranteed that the drug would not be abused. Lauding these rigorous controls set by the Japanese, Mohnike drew attention to the opium addiction prevalent among the Chinese at their colony adjoining Dejima: "The children of the Celestial Empire living in the Chinese trading post at Nagasaki abandon themselves to this beloved passion perhaps even more than they do in their motherland."[30]

The traditional extended-family system with its veneration of the elderly provided strong assurance of adequate care for the aging. There were no institutions for the old or for invalids, no infirmaries, and no orphanages. To ensure that the family tradition was in fact followed, the law required that the next of kin care for the elderly and the indigent sick. As a further protective measure, larger communities paid an annual retainer to at least one practitioner, usually an acupuncturist, for which he in turn dispensed free medical care to any indigent sick who sought his help. The government made similar services available to sick prisoners. Although these regulations and services were theoretically valid, Mohnike judged, on the evidence of the large numbers of beggars and imploring lepers on the Tokaido, that the law was not enforced.

The government's approach to the possibility of famine contrasted sharply with its general laxity toward many other aspects of public health. Rice furnished the major staple of the Japanese diet; the availability and consumption of wheat was limited. Rice crops, Mohnike was told, were more susceptible to failure than those of any other grain. To guard against such disaster, the government had erected a considerable number of storehouses throughout the empire and stocked these with rice and wheat equal in amount to a full year's harvest. Mohnike viewed this program as a largely political exercise: widespread famine would undoubtedly incite a

[29]Mohnike, "Aanteekeningen over de Geneeskunde der Japanezen," p. 234.
[30]Ibid., p. 237.

rebellion, in the course of which, he predicted, the people would overthrow the shogunate and establish intercourse with the family of Western nations.[31]

Smallpox was probably introduced into Japan by the crews of Korean trading vessels in the seventh century, and the first recorded epidemic occurred in A.D. 735. The disease became endemic with periodic epidemics; one of these was rampant when Mohnike arrived at Dejima in 1848.

The Japanese believed that smallpox was a visitation from the gods and that all human beings were destined to be afflicted. Some attributed it to an internal toxin that interacted with an extrinsic poison. The lower classes blamed smallpox on a devil-god whose evil workings could be thwarted by witchcraft, among other means. They dedicated small shrines to this malignant deity, and in the Fukuoka fief people hung wood-block prints and posters of *Bamboo Saizo,* a doll with a branch of bamboo in his hand and a monkey at his side, in order to repel the smallpox devil.

The Chinese also accepted smallpox as a divinely instituted punishment, and for this reason they termed the disease the "Heavenly Flowers." Chinese practitioners were using inoculation (also variolation) as early as A.D. 1000. By introducing the disease from a mild or convalescent case, they produced an immunity that was, at times, only temporary. The method was to implant powdered crusts in the nostril or ear by inserting a goose feather or puffing a pipe—into the right nostril or ear of a boy, and the left of a girl. Or they soaked fluid from a pox on a plug of cloth and inserted it in a similar manner. A third procedure was to have the subject wear the contaminated undergarments of a victim of the disease, preferably a child. A similar method was used in India by Brahmin priests affiliated with the cult of the smallpox deity.

Inoculation by a more direct method was practiced in Turkey, originally to protect the Circassian beauties of the seraglios. Fluid from a mature pox was rubbed into one or more scarified areas on the arm. What was probably the first extensive description of the technique was forwarded to Western Europe in December 1713 by Emanuel Timoni, a graduate of Padua, then practicing in Constantinople. He sent it to John Woodward, a London physician who read the communication to the Royal Society, of which Timoni was a member; it appeared in the society's *Philosophical Transactions* in 1714 and 1716.

A few years later, Lady Mary Wortley Montagu (1689-1762) became the outspoken and victorious champion of inoculation for Western Europe. She had suffered a severe case of smallpox in London in December 1715 that left her face heavily pitted and with no eyelashes. The following September, she came to Constantinople with her husband, Edward, who was the new ambassador to the Ottoman Porte. Lady Mary observed the

---

[31] For a corrective to Mohnike's point of view, see Hugh Borton, *Peasant Uprisings in Japan in the Tokugawa Period* (New York: Paragon, 1968).

technique at Adrianople and in March 1718 had her son inoculated by the embassy surgeon. Upon her return to London, she pressed vigorously for inoculation, but only after several years of controversy did the English accept its value.

The Chinese method of inoculation was introduced into Japan in the middle of the eighteenth century, when Li Jen Shan (also Rijinsan), a Chinese who had moved to Japan, first performed the technique on twenty children in Nagasaki. At the end of the century, L. A. Bernard Keller, a doctor at Dejima, inoculated six children using the Turkish technique. Four of these attempts were successful. When Keller visited Edo in 1794 on the *hofreis,* he instructed the *Rangakusha* in the method of inoculation, and Otsuki Gentaku and other *Rangakusha* are said to have applied it to protect members of their families. Of the two techniques, the Chinese was the more favored, probably because it did not scarify the human body. Ogata Shunsaku of Fukuoka fief and Nagayo Shuntatsu (or Toshitatsu) of Omura performed inoculations and trained students. The Omura clan also established three *shutozan* (inoculation mountains) for the isolation of smallpox victims.

It was not until the end of the eighteenth century that completely effective protection against smallpox was discovered. Within one decade, vaccination circumnavigated the world and entered every major country, save Japan. Edward Jenner (1749-1823), a country practitioner in Gloucestershire, England, recognized that the dairy maids in his shire contracted cowpox while milking animals, and thereby became immune to smallpox. On May 14, 1796, he performed the first vaccination against smallpox, using cowpox.

The European powers were eager to introduce vaccination into their colonies, scourged by smallpox. It was through these efforts that vaccination ultimately reached Japan. It came to China in 1805, following a route from Spain through Spanish America and the Philippines. The way to Japan was more complex: from Vienna to Constantinople, to Baghdad, Basra, Bombay, the French colonies Réunion and Ile de France in the Indian Ocean, to Batavia, and finally in 1849 to Nagasaki, after repeated attempts had failed owing to the *Bakufu's* ban on the entry of foreign children.

Jean de Carro (1770-1856) was responsible for the dissemination of smallpox vaccination in Europe and the Near East. The historian Sigerist describes him as "a great promoter and salesman. . . . He never made a discovery himself, but he usually showed good judgment in taking up other people's findings."[32]

Born in Geneva, Carro studied medicine at Edinburgh from 1790 to 1793 but then chose to practice in Vienna because the French Revolution

[32]Letters of Jean de Carro to Alexandre Marcet, 1794-1822, H. E. Sigerist, ed. Supplements to the *Bulletin of the History of Medicine,* no. 12 (Baltimore: The Johns Hopkins Press, 1950), pp. 2-3.

had made Geneva so politically turbulent. He obtained threads impregnated with Jenner's vaccine from Alexandre Marcet (1770-1822), a leading physician and lecturer in chemistry at Guy's Hospital in London. Carro performed the first successful vaccination in Vienna on April 29 or 30, 1799, upon the son of a physician.

The Asian journey of vaccination began in the summer of 1800, at a formal banquet given by Lord Minto, the British ambassador to Austria. The guests included Carro and Mr. and Mrs. Nisbet, who were on their way to Constantinople to visit their pregnant daughter, the wife of Thomas Bruce, Lord Elgin, ambassador to Turkey. Carro extolled to the Nisbets the benefits of vaccination and particularly its importance for infants.

When the Nisbets arrived in Constantinople, they relayed to the Elgins Carro's comments on the virtues of vaccination, and in September 1800 Carro received a request from Lord Elgin for vaccine for his own son. The first lymph Carro sent was inert when it reached Constantinople, but the second specimen was viable. The Elgins now became ardent champions of vaccination; Lady Elgin vaccinated children in the foreign community and made the technique available to physicians from Western Europe practicing there.

The introduction of vaccination to India, where hundreds of thousands were maimed or died from smallpox, now became the goal of Lord Elgin and Carro. Efforts to send vaccine from England to Bombay via the Cape of Good Hope route, a voyage of 10,500 nautical miles, were unsuccessful. At Jenner's suggestion, youths were recruited for the voyage and vaccinated serially in order to preserve the lymph. Previous failure had been attributed to "the odor of the pitch." On another occasion, the East India Company sent the *Queen* to Bombay with vaccine, but she foundered at the Cape of Good Hope. In March 1801, the Honorable John Duncan, governor of Bombay, asked Lord Elgin to send vaccine from Basra. Situated at the head of the Persian Gulf, Basra was only 1,500 nautical miles from Bombay.

At this time, Carro began to use lymph prepared by Dr. Luigi Sacco of Varese, Lombardy. The Italian had obtained it from cows at a fair in Lugano, and forwarded a supply to Carro in 1801. It was probably a more durable strain than the Jenner-Woodville, which Carro had been using, and it was Sacco's lymph that Carro supplied for the shipment to Bombay. As Carro commented, "Great Britain supplied the Occident and the Republic of Italy, the Orient."[33] At Lord Elgin's request, Sacco's lymph was forwarded to Baghdad, where a Dr. Milne, the physician attached to the British embassy, used it for several vaccinations to heighten its virulence before shipment to Bombay. The first shipment failed, but the second was successful, and in June 1802, the first vaccination was performed on the subcontinent. The subject was Anna Dusthall, an Anglo-Indian child whose father was a servant to a British military officer.

[33] J. de Carro, *Histoire de la vaccination en Turque et Grèce et aux Indes Orientales.* Sciences et Arts, 6e année, t. 18 (Genève, 1801), p. 343.

From Bombay, the passage to the French colony Ile de France and Réunion in the Indian Ocean was the next leg of the voyage of vaccination to Japan. M. Laborde, a physician on Ile de France, made repeated but unsuccessful efforts to obtain viable lymph from both France and England. Success finally came about in 1803 through the use of human subjects: "A French captain, coming from India, had the good fortune to preserve the virus fresh by successive vaccinations made from arm to arm during the voyage."[34]

The Dutch made several efforts to introduce vaccination into Japan, but the obstacle here was the Japanese interdict against admitting children. Several efforts failed on the six-week August voyage through the torrid, tropical waters. At last, in 1849, forty-five years after vaccination had reached Batavia, capillary tubes filled with smallpox scabs and fluid from pox arrived at Dejima in a viable state.

The first Japanese to learn the actual technique of vaccination, Nakagawa Goroji, had been seized in 1807 on a small northern Japanese island by the crew of a Russian ship. After his release on the Russian coast, he spent several years wandering across Siberia and there learned the technique of vaccination. In 1812, Nakagawa returned to Kunashirijima, another northern island, with two Russian pamphlets on vaccination against smallpox.

The following year, Baba Sadayoshi (also Sajuro), a Dutch interpreter on Hokkaido, learned Russian from the Russian captain Golowin, who was being held in detention there. His ship, a fighting sloop, had been seized by the Japanese in 1811 while Golowin was appraising the coastlines of Hokkaido and the Kuriles. Baba translated Nakagawa's smallpox pamphlets into Japanese. For some reason, Baba hid the translation in his clothes box until 1820, when it appeared under the title *Tonka Hiketsu.*

Several Japanese practitioners, who had studied Dutch books on the use of cowpox, endeavored to initiate vaccination into Japan. Nagayo Toshitatsu (or Shuntatsu), of Hizen in Omura, purchased two cows infected with cowpox and tried to vaccinate babies; no information is available as to the outcome of his efforts. Koyama Shisei of Kishu kumano and Minakami Sotan of Sanuki also made early efforts to vaccinate: they attempted to transfer human smallpox lymph to cows and then to use the fluid from the resultant lesions as vaccine.

Nabeshima Kanzo (1814-1871) of Saga, also of Hizen, learned of vaccination, and at his request Mohnike instructed Narabayashi Soken, an interpreter, in the technique.[35] Nabeshima also asked Mohnike in 1848 to obtain lymph from Batavia, but it was inert when it reached Dejima.

---

[34] His report is contained in a letter to the *Philadelphia Medical and Surgical Journal,* 1806, *2:* 71-75.

[35] As *daimyo* of Hizen, Nabeshima had the duty of protecting Nagasaki from foreign invasion and so became interested in Western technology. In 1850 he had the first reverberatory furnace built, with Dutch technical assistance.

Success came the following year, when after Mohnike obtained live vaccine Narabayashi was able to vaccinate the son of Nabeshima as well as his own boy. Nabeshima then launched a campaign to proclaim vaccination; he had color posters prepared showing how he had allowed the use of the procedure on his own son. They were circulated across his fief to persuade his subjects to submit to vaccination. Another *tozama daimyo,* Shimazu Nariakira, the lord of Satsuma fief, not only promoted vaccination in his *han* but also sent lymph to the Ryuku Islands, which he considered his domain.

Mohnike's most rewarding opportunity to learn about Japan came—as it had for many of his predecessors in the post at Dejima—when he accompanied Levijssohn, the *opperhoofd,* on the *hofreis* to Edo. They left Nagasaki in the winter of 1849 and returned in June of that year. The *hofreis* had begun as an annual event, but after 1790 it became a quadrennial trip because of the steadily declining profits of the Dutch trade. The 120-day journey gave Mohnike a chance to visit and learn about Miyako, the beautiful old capital, and to see the shogun's seat of power at Edo. Many Japanese doctors sought Mohnike's advice about their cases and even brought patients to the roadside for him to evaluate.

In the summer of 1850, Mohnike left Dejima for assignments at Borneo and Batavia. In 1853 he published his extensive observations on the practice of medicine and the introduction of vaccination in Japan, in the first number of the *Geneeskundig Tijdschrift voor Nederlandsch-Indië.* He then investigated the culture and flora and fauna of the islands; he published the results after his return to Germany.[36]

Mohnike was promoted to the rank of medical officer, first class, in January 1855, and to supervisory medical officer, second class, and inspector of hospitals in December 1862. His work during a major outbreak of cholera and, later, of malaria, brought promotion to the rank of supervisory medical officer, first class.

Mohnike retired in October 1869 and returned to Germany, where he published further material on the Japanese.[37] On January 26, 1887, he died at Bonn.

[36]Otto Mohnike, *Banka und Palembang nebst Mittheilungen ueber Sumatra in Allgemeinen* (Münster, 1874); *Ueber geschwänzte Menschen* (Münster, 1878); *Blicke auf das Pflanzen- und Tierleben in den niederländischen Malaienländer* (Münster, 1883).

[37]Otto Mohnike, *Die Japaner: Eine ethnogr. Monographie* (Münster, 1872); "Volksaberglauben: Legenden und Ueberlieferungen der Japaner" in *Globus, 1872, 21.*

3

J. K. van den Broek and
the Rise of Technology in Japan

After Jan Karel van den Broek (1814-1865) succeeded Mohnike in August 1853, the focus of studies at Dejima shifted from medicine and natural history to chemistry, physics, and technology. This was the result of a felicitous combination of interests. Van den Broek was knowledgeable in those fields, and several of the *tozama daimyo* were eager to develop Western industries, primarily those having a military application. In 1855, twenty Dutchmen began to teach naval tactics at Nagasaki. Students from Kyushu and from the *Bakufu* itself studied at the naval school with Van den Broek.[1]

Born in 1814, Van den Broek trained in surgery at the clinical school in Rotterdam until 1833, when he joined the Corps of Royal Rifles and was posted in Arnhem. He showed an early interest in physics by publishing, in 1842, two papers on auditory mechanics.[2]

In January 1852 a notice requesting applicants for six medical posts in Java appeared in *Nederlandsche Staatscourant,* with preference to be given to those who were doctors of medicine, surgery, or obstetrics; Van den Broek's petition was accepted in March of that year. After his arrival in Batavia, he practiced in North Java and in May 1853 was appointed physician at Dejima. The following month, the responsibilities attached to the appointment were expanded to include research in natural science.

Van den Broek's lectures in natural science attracted representatives of the shogun's court. The lessons culminated in a display of the new electromagnetic telegraph, and he was asked to make a model for the court in Edo. Van den Broek's demonstrations—for example, of a wooden model of a steam engine, naval fortifications, and the telegraph—continued

---

[1]See J. MacLean, "The significance of Jan Karel van den Broek (1814-1865) for the introduction of Western technology into Japan," *Japanese Studies in the History of Science,* 1977, *16:* 69-90.

[2]J. K. van den Broek, "Iets over de schuinische plaatsing van het Trommelvlies en over de mechanische werking der Gehoorbeentjes bij het hooren," *Algemeene Kunst-en Letterbode,* vol. 1 (Haarlem, 1842), pp. 106-9. "Beschrijving van eenen nieuwen Oorspiegel (Speculum Auris), ibid., vol. 2 (1842), pp. 34-37, 42. Van den Broek subsequently used *Natuurkundig Schoolboek* as the principal text for his classes in Nagasaki. The first steam engine, completed by the Japanese in 1856, was a copy of an illustration in Timmer's text. MacLean, "Significance of Jan Karel van den Broek," pp. 70-71.

to draw Japanese scholars to Dejima. When the *Soembing,* commanded by Gerhardus Fabius (1806-88), arrived in Nagasaki in 1854, it carried an electromagnetic telegraph as a gift from King Willem III to the shogun. The telegraph had been damaged on the high seas, and Van den Broek was able to repair it.[3]

By 1855, Van den Broek was giving classes on telegraphy, steam engines, iron foundries, and shipbuilding, as well as other technological subjects. At the request of several *tozama daimyo,* he made wooden models of blast furnaces for them to copy. He also taught young men from Hizen about dock construction and the most suitable types of wood for such projects. As his reputation grew, students came from as far away as Mito fief, northeast of Edo.[4]

Although technology was his major concentration, Van den Broek continued to be active in medicine. From the time of his arrival, he was hailed in the lanes of Nagasaki as "the Dejima doctor," and sick people, some of whom had come from a distance, stopped him for consultation. The interpreters also discussed their patients with him, and practitioners sought his advice on the few, superficial surgical procedures they undertook. In further recognition of the mounting interest in technology, in December 1855, at the request of the Nagasaki *bugyo,* Okabe Suruga, Van den Broek added to his classes for the Nagasaki interpreters instruction in arithmetic, geometry, chemistry, and physics. The popularity of Western medicine was further attested to in 1856, when the shogunate sent 150 students to Van den Broek for instruction. In his last year at Nagasaki, five Kyushu *daimyo* sent gifts to Van den Broek to honor his contributions in technology. In that year his enrollment had swelled to a total of 264 students.

Despite his popularity as an instructor and consultant, Rear Admiral G.C.C. Pels Rycken (1810-89) reported to Batavia that Van den Broek was increasingly abrasive in his behavior toward the Japanese. He drew the ire of the Dutch authorities by making unpatriotic statements in letters to Java newspapers. Donker Curtius, appointed *opperhoofd* in 1852, decided that he was impeding the furtherance of friendly relations with the Japanese, and Van den Broek was given an honorable discharge in October 1857. He returned to the Netherlands, an embittered man, and died there in May 1865.

Commodore Matthew Perry's successful expedition in 1853 convinced the Japanese of the lamentable state of their defenses. One of their first

---

[3] MacLean quotes a letter from Gerhardus Fabius to Van den Broek, dated 23 October 1854, wishing him success in his efforts to teach technology to the Japanese, thirsty for such information. Fabius added that Van den Broek would be recorded then as a major benefactor in the annals of Japanese history. MacLean, "Significance of Jan Karel van den Broek," p. 94. See also *Kolonien,* 15 June 1859, ¶: 839.

[4] Mito fief was particularly important as one of the three branches from which the Tokugawa shogun could be chosen.

acts in response to this recognition was the decision to develop a navy, and they applied to the opperhoofd, Donker Curtius, for assistance. He suggested that they ask for a detachment of naval officers to teach naval science and technology; he also asked The Hague to send a frigate with such a detachment. In answer to Curtius's request, The Hague sent the frigate *Soembing* to Japan. In 1855 the Netherlands gave the *Soembing* to the *Bakufu,* and she was renamed *Kanko Maru,* the first fighting ship in the Japanese navy.

As a Dutch doctor who came to Dejima two years later commented, the Japanese had been the dupes of a Trojan horse, for no sooner had the naval detachment arrived than Curtius insisted that since they had come at the invitation of the Japanese, they should not be so confined as their predecessors had been. The Japanese consented to this proposal and extended their grant to all the Dutch on Dejima. Thus, after two centuries, the gates of Dejima opened and its residents could at last move freely in and out.

Following Van den Broek's dismissal, the *Bakufu* decided that they wanted a Dutch doctor at Dejima whose main responsibility would be to teach medicine on a more regular basis than previously, with the collaboration of the government. For the post, the commander of the Dutch naval detachment, W. J. C. Ridder Huyssen Kattendyke, chose Johannes Lydius Catherinus Pompe van Meerdervoort, a twenty-nine-year-old doctor who, although he had never taught before, turned out to be ideally suited for the task. It is the good fortune of modern students of the period that Pompe's own journal furnishes an extensive and perceptive commentary on the years he spent in Japan: what he saw, learned, and accomplished there.[5]

Pompe van Meerdervoort was born May 5, 1829, in Bruges, the beautiful Flemish capital, at one time the busiest seaport of northern Europe. Descended from a military family, he entered the military medical school at Utrecht in 1846. After graduation in 1849, he was assigned to service in the East Indies naval forces for six years and returned to Holland in 1856, when Huyssen van Kattendyke made him his appointee. The mission sailed in March 1857 and, after a stopover at Batavia, reached Dejima in September.

When Pompe sailed for Japan, he had envisaged no larger role for himself than that of the Dejima doctor—by tradition both a physician and a teacher. ". . . it had not escaped the attention of the Japanese government that a number of Nagasaki doctors had made a national reputation and had shown by successful medical practice that they really knew more than their Japanese colleagues."[6] But after he had been at Dejima for a brief period, Pompe decided to set up a full-fledged course of medical instruction. He

[5] See *Doctor on Desima,* translated and annotated by Elizabeth P. Wittermans and John Z. Bowers (Tokyo: Sophia University, 1970).
[6] Ibid., p. 84.

was influenced in part by his conclusion "that the needs of the Japanese were much greater than had been assumed. . . . the rational basis of their knowledge was zero and they had derived only very inexact ideas from the Dutch medical literature."[7] Furthermore, Pompe was an ambitious and talented young man, and he perceived here an opportunity to advance the state of medicine in Japan and at the same time advance his own career.

It was first necessary to obtain the cooperation of the Japanese officials at Nagasaki. By a stroke of luck, this came about easily through the intercession of Pompe's first medical student, Matsumoto Ryojun (1832-1907). He was the son of a distinguished physician, Sato Taizen, and after serving an apprenticeship with his father had become one of the physicians attached to the shogunate as *Omemie-ishi* (physician with the honor of attending the shogun). But Matsumoto's heart was set on studying at Nagasaki, and his arrival there coincided with Pompe's. They agreed that Matsumoto would supervise the students and serve as their intermediary with Pompe, while proceeding at the same time with his own studies. Pompe admired him greatly as a man of common sense and exceptional talent. With Matsumoto's help, Pompe's study of Japanese progressed rapidly: after a few months he noticed that the students could understand much of what he said as long as he spoke slowly and enunciated clearly.[8]

The five-year medical curriculum began with instruction in biology, chemistry, and physics. Lectures and demonstrations in the basic medical sciences followed. The first class, numbering twelve in all, was drawn from the court at Edo and the *tozama* fiefs on Kyushu. Other students came to the school to learn geology, mineralogy, physics, and chemistry. They were joined by students from the gunnery school and apprentices from the school for mechanical arts. As a result, Pompe found his teaching load even larger, but he was surprised and pleased at the diligence and aptitude of his willing learners: "During the classes they were very attentive, and they continued to ask questions until they understood everything well."[9] In turn, Pompe exercised the patience required of a good teacher and made sure that he was doing all he could to answer their questions and their needs—as he states in his memoirs.

It was clear to Pompe that the mere teaching of theory was insufficient to promote real knowledge. Since dissection was banned, he was forced to rely for practical instruction in anatomy on cutting up the heads of cows and on a few old anatomical charts, until after one year a pâpier-maché

[7] Ibid.

[8] By comparison with Matsumoto, Pompe found most of the interpreters intolerable. When one of them came to him drunk and claimed that he had a message from the Nagasaki *bugyo*, Pompe handled the situation with dispatch: "He refused to leave and became uncouth. . . . I threw him very calmly down a flight of stairs (twenty of them) and out into the street." Ibid., p. 25.

[9] Ibid., p. 86.

model arrived from Paris. It was not until two years after the opening of the school and repeated requests that approval finally came from Edo for Pompe to perform an autopsy.

Up to this point, examinations of corpses had consisted merely of dismemberments by untrained *eta*. On September 9, 1859, Pompe made the first professional post-mortem examination in Japan. Since the government would not allow a public building to be defiled, the procedure had to be carried out in a hastily erected shed, which was demolished as soon as the autopsy had been completed. In addition to the medical students, twenty-four practitioners were granted permits to attend.

Another Japanese tradition that Pompe perceived as pernicious was that of class distinctions made in the health services that doctors could provide and patients receive. He was to some extent able to challenge that custom by making it known that his own services were available to all who needed them.[10]

Pompe had also made repeated requests for a teaching hospital, but again two years elapsed before approval came from the *Bakufu*. Pompe's heroic efforts to control a devastating cholera epidemic during the summer of 1858 persuaded the Japanese to respond favorably to his petitions. The teaching hospital, Yojosho ("preservation of health"), opened on September 21, 1861, with 120 beds. A new medical-school building that housed a lecture hall, seminar/demonstration rooms, and student dormitories adjoined it.

Pompe's back-breaking schedule now included his responsibilities as sole physician for the hospital and as instructor of all the subjects in the medical curriculum. To his lectures came increasing numbers of practicing physicians, attired in their traditional robes and hairstyle and carrying a single sword. Behind each physician knelt his assistant, bearing on his back the practitioner's portable dispensary. Occasionally an unlicensed practitioner joined the class.

Pompe's tenure in Japan was closely tied to that of his friend the *opperhoofd* Donker Curtius. When the latter returned to Holland in 1860, his successor, Mr. J. K. DeWit, proved a disappointment to Pompe, who ascribed to him the declining reputation of the Netherlands in Japan. This feeling, compounded by fatigue, caused him to advise the Japanese authorities at the beginning of 1862 that he would himself return to the Netherlands by the end of that year.

DeWit then caused further vexation, in connection with the question of Pompe's successor. Pompe, fearful that the British would take over, was determined to see the medical school and hospital continue under Dutch leadership, and he accordingly proposed Dr. C. G. Mansvelt, then serving in the Dutch navy, who had impressed Pompe when his ship visited

[10]Ibid., p. 90.

Nagasaki in 1860. DeWit was evidently unconcerned as to the future of the school, and his relations with Pompe had deteriorated to the extent that he rejected the recommendation out of hand.

Pompe then proposed another compatriot, Dr. Antonius François Bauduin (1822-1885); the latter's appointment was secured. Bauduin, a military medical officer, had been teaching medicine at Pompe's former school in Utrecht for more than twelve years. He arrived in Dejima in September 1862 and assumed Pompe's responsibilities the following month.

Shortly before his departure, Pompe awarded diplomas to sixty-one students, whom he ranked in three categories: those who were fully qualified to practice medicine, those who had performed only satisfactorily, and those who were not qualified to treat patients without supervision. Among Pompe's graduates were men who became leaders in medicine. Doi Shunzo was an excellent anatomist and wrote a popular handbook on that subject; Hashimoto Tsunatsune founded the Japanese Red Cross hospital system; and Nagayo Sensai was a key figure in the early years of Meiji medicine. Two medical students, Ito Hosei and Hayashi Kenkai, who had been selected to continue their studies in the Netherlands, accompanied Pompe when he left.

As Pompe was preparing to sail, on November 1, 1862, the Nagasaki *bugyo* sent a high-ranking officer to confer a formal farewell accolade. Pompe was deeply touched when he noticed, as his ship left the bay, that the Dutch flag was flying side by side with the Japanese flag over the hospital—a symbol of the strong and enduring bonds that he had established with the Japanese.

Under Bauduin's leadership, the school, now known as Seitokukan (May 1865), expanded and strengthened its educational programs and facilities. As the number of students preparing for careers in technology and industry increased, chemistry, physics, and mathematics were made a separate curriculum. In keeping with the growing Japanese emphasis on industrialization and military might, technical applications were stressed. The *bugyo,* Hattori Saemonnosuke, and the *Bakufu* reinforced this trend by supplying funds for the appointment of a teacher and to provide facilities for the new program. Koenraad Wolter Gratama (1831-1888), a Dutch chemist, came to Nagasaki in May 1866 to fill the new post.

Gratama, a very methodical man, kept a diary from the day he left Utrecht, in February 1866; unfortunately, the diaries of the years in Nagasaki are unavailable. But Gratama was also an avid correspondent, and his letters provide a revealing portrait of the life-style of a Dutch teacher at Nagasaki in 1866.[11]

Gratama was cordially received by Antonius Bauduin:

[11]I am indebted to Jan Eggink, the husband of Gratama's granddaughter, for making excerpts from Gratama's letters available to me.

My principal, Bauduin, had already straightened up my room; he helps with everything and is still looking out for my needs. The first days, he invited me for dinner, pretending that I was too cramped for space to eat comfortably in my lodgings.[12]

Soon after he settled in Nagasaki, Gratama wrote a picturesque account of one of his typical days in that torrid city:

I shall now describe my life in Nagasaki. The time to get up in the morning is fixed at seven, and usually the undersigned appears some time later, dressed in East Indian night dress, consisting of night trousers and *cabaya,* only to lie down again in an easy chair placed before the open window. The Japanese boy has made tea earlier, and I am hardly seated before he comes and offers me a cup of good Chinese tea. Although in Nagasaki we live amidst big tea plantations growing a kind that is considered in Japan to be very good, the Europeans never take Japanese tea.

At about ten o'clock the conflict begins between the attraction of work at the hospital and that of the easy chair. Usually that fight does not last long before the sense of duty takes the side of the hospital.

With a straw hat on the head and a Japanese parasol in the hand, I start the trip to the hospital through the blazing heat of Nagasaki and then up the steep hill. In the street one can easily study Japanese home life, because in such heat everything that can be opened is flung wide. I believe that for this purpose the women even open their sewing boxes! After a quarter of an hour I arrive at the hospital.

Gratama goes on to describe the facilities and his teaching schedule:

Three buildings belong to the hospital: the biggest one contains the wards and the dispensary, the second is the dormitory for about forty students, and the third is my building. It is oblong and one-storied, with a porch all around. It is a new building and looks rather well, both inside and outside. It contains eight rooms all giving onto a central corridor.

In the laboratory I usually find some ten students, most of them twenty-five to forty years old or more. They all understand some Dutch, some of them very well, but they have difficulty in speaking it. I take half an hour or one hour for tiffin while the students continue their laboratory work. At about 3:30 my lecture begins and is translated by one of the students into Japanese. It lasts till 5:30, and then I have earned my pay.[13]

In the spring of 1867, the Japanese government decided that Gratama's school should be transferred to Edo, where it became Kaiseisho:

This is a wide tract in Yedo on which are located schools for teaching European science. One could compare it with our academies, *mutatis mutandis,* of course. Previously, European languages and chemistry were taught here. There is a printing

[12]Letter, 13 May 1866.
[13]Letter, 29 July 1866.

plant (European), collections of books, stones, insects, etc., and a botanical garden, all of which are very primitive. Up to a few years ago this school had another name, i.e., 'the place where the books of barbarians are read.' Since the arrival of the Europeans, the natives have learned to distinguish between a better civilization and a lack of civilization, and the Japanese have come to the conclusion that they themselves were the barbarians.[14]

Because reactionary elements continued to hate the foreigners, fifteen Japanese soldiers guarded the school, and a detachment accompanied Gratama when he walked the streets. As an added protection, he carried a revolver, a pistol, and a rifle.

Construction of Gratama's new teaching laboratory had been switched to the site of two warehouses. He drew up the necessary plans, but the Japanese proceeded slowly, and he wrote that his teaching program would not start for at least six months: "Everything is done slowly in Japan, and the Japanese usually tell the foreigners so."[15] He discarded the possibility of practicing medicine in the meantime:

Moreover, it can be only a consultative practice, because up to now we are not permitted to make house calls. My greatest objection to practicing is that the Japanese are too poor to pay the golden fee for a visit—two or three dollars. Usually they give a chicken or eggs. In Nagasaki, practice among the Japanese yielded no more than effusions of gratitude. I already have such a big stock of those that I can live on them for the next few years.[16]

The fighting between the imperial armies and the Tokugawa forces in the spring of 1868 made it necessary for Gratama to take refuge at the residence of the Netherlands consul in Yokohama.

Meanwhile, development of a proper library marked further advancement in the Nagasaki school's progress. This was facilitated by an augmented flow of European books, which now reached Nagasaki within one year of their publication in Holland. A small printing press was installed at Dejima, so that teaching manuals could be readily reproduced. The teaching program in gynecology, one of Bauduin's special interests, was expanded and a well-equipped surgical unit established.

The large number of patients with eye diseases prompted Bauduin to designate a ward for them. He was the first to use the ophthalmoscope routinely and greatly improved the treatment of squint and trachoma. He instructed his students in the safe and effective use of potentially dangerous silver nitrate and carbolic acid for inflammatory eye disorders. Unskilled practitioners used these substances extensively, but often in amounts that worsened the problem.

[14]Letter, 9 June 1867.
[15]Letter, 29 July 1866.
[16]Letter, 24 August 1868.

In June 1865, Bauduin sent a message to the *Bakufu* stating that four of the medical students whom they had sent to Nagasaki wished to continue their studies in Europe. However, he would recommend only one of them, Ogata Kosai. When several months passed without a response, in September 1866 Bauduin and Gratama went to Edo to explain to the *Bakufu* the advantages of study in Europe. Further support for Ogata's request was provided by the Dutch minister, D. de Graff van Poelsbrock, who had transferred his embassy from Dejima to Yokohama in order to be with the other foreign representatives. He volunteered free passage for Ogata to Holland, but the *Bakufu*, still fearful of Western contacts, refused.

In January 1867, Bauduin decided to return to Europe for postgraduate studies in gynecology and recommended as his successor C. G. Mansvelt, the man whom Pompe van Meerdervoort had in vain proposed for the post just two years earlier. But now there was no need to go through Dutch-governmental channels, and approval came promptly from the *Bakufu*.[17]

With Mansvelt firmly settled as his successor, Bauduin booked passage for Holland in February 1867. As the day of his departure approached, the *bugyo* told him that the *Bakufu* had finally relented and awarded Ogata a scholarship for study in Europe. (The one-and-a-half-year delay in granting Bauduin's request was another example of the *Bakufu*'s vacillation on contacts with the West.) Ogata enrolled at Utrecht, but with the fall of the *Bakufu* on November 9, 1867, his financial support ceased, and he returned to Japan in March 1870.

In July 1869 Gratama wrote that he had moved to Osaka, where he was teaching chemistry and physics. The following year he returned to The Hague. Meanwhile, Bauduin was completing postgraduate studies in gynecological surgery with Professor Sir Thomas Wells (1818-1897), an expert in ovariotomy at St. Thomas's Hospital in London. At the request of the *Bakufu*, he drew up plans for a naval hospital at Edo. Bauduin set out for Japan in 1868, but the fighting that attended the fall of the shogunate obliged him to wait in Shanghai until May 1869. After a period at Nagasaki, he moved to a hospital on the grounds of the affluent Daifukuji temple in Osaka. Here he pioneered in introducing ovariotomy to Japan. He also assisted in the founding at Osaka of the first military medical school and hospital.

Bauduin spent several months of 1870 as adviser on the development of a medical school in Okayama City, southwest of Osaka. In November of that year, he decided to leave Japan permanently. He had guided the Nagasaki medical school into a new educational role in chemistry and physics, he had pioneered in ophthalmology and gynecology, and he had proven himself to be a worthy successor to Pompe van Meerdervoort.

[17]Mansvelt, after his earlier rejection as Pompe's successor, had returned to Holland and resigned his naval commission. But he possessed an abiding love for the Orient and returned to Shanghai, where he opened a medical clinic and pharmacy.

Just as he was about to leave Japan, Bauduin was persuaded to spend a few months teaching medicine at Toko, the medical school in Tokyo. (The Prussian medical mission that had been designated to introduce German medicine there had been delayed by the Franco-Prussian War.) He did so, and then in 1872 returned to the Netherlands, where he died on June 2, 1885.

The collapse of the Bakufu and the flight of the Nagasaki *bugyo* severely disrupted the medical school at Nagasaki. Many of the students became "lost souls." Some decided to return to their homes in the Kanto and Kansai regions, and a few went to the extreme of booking passage for Shanghai on the American ship S.S. *Costa Rica.* However, Ambassador van Poelsbrock urged the new government to retain Mansvelt and continue the program at the school; fortunately, they heeded his advice. A measure of stability was restored to the Nagasaki school on June 21, 1868, with the appointment of Nagayo Sensai, Pompe's most able student, as director.

In the fall of 1868, Inoue Kaoru (1836-1915), of the Choshu clan, came to Nagasaki as a senior official of the Meiji government and gave further assurances as to the continuation of the school. He announced that henceforth it would be known as Nagasaki-fu Igakko and that the teaching hospital would continue to be affiliated with it. With the introduction of *gunken-seido,* the prefectural system, in 1871, responsibilities for the school passed to Nagasaki prefecture, and the name was changed accordingly to Nagasaki-ken Igakko.

In the spring of that year, Mansvelt decided to seek a new position. Yoshio Keisai, the administrative officer of *Igakko,* was serving as adviser to the progressive Kumamoto prefecture, which was developing a medical school and hospital. On his recommendation, Mansvelt headed the Kumamoto medical school from 1871 to 1874. His restlessness sent him on to hospitals with medical training programs in Kyoto (1876 to 1878) and in Osaka (1879). From there, he returned to the Netherlands, where he died at The Hague in 1912.

Dr. Van Leeuwen van Duivenbode succeeded Mansvelt at Nagasaki, and Dr. Christiaan Jacob Ermerins (1841-1880) from Osaka joined him as the second member of the teaching staff. In June 1879 Dr. Cornelius Hendricus Matheus Fock (1845-1883) replaced Van Duivenbode.

4

William Willis

The final stages of more than two centuries of rule by the Tokugawa shogunate began in the summer of 1858, when the American envoy, Townsend Harris (1804-1878), signed a commercial treaty between Japan and the United States.[1] At that time, only two isolated ports were open: Hakodate, on the northern island of Hokkaido, and Shimoda, southwest of Edo. The treaty called for four ports: Nagasaki; Niigata, on the Japan Sea; Kanagawa, south of Edo; and Hyogo, near Osaka. Import and export duties were established, American citizens were granted extraterritoriality, and the bans on Christianity were eased.

The impact of the treaty on the Japanese mood was profound. The majority of the people could not tolerate the presence of the *Namban* ("Southern barbarians"), whom for centuries they had been taught to detest. Thus, foreigners lived in constant jeopardy, and physical attacks—including murders—were not uncommon.

America soon became involved in her Civil War and so could not take advantage of her favorable position as the nation that "opened" Japan. Instead, Britain became the dominant Western power in Japan, with France in second place. England's first venture in Japan, a trading post on Hirado Island, had been a dismal failure: it was closed after one decade because of poor management and what one loyal Englishman called "ruthless competition from the Dutch."[2] But when Perry opened Japan, Britain, with her far-flung empire, was the greatest world power. Her government was stable under a parliamentary system and a constitutional monarch, Queen Victoria, who had reigned since 1837.

It seemed only natural for Britain, as the most firmly established imperialist power in China, to seek a comparable position in Japan. She also regarded Japan as a further vantage point from which to watch Russian efforts in the Far East. James Bruce Elgin, eighth earl of Elgin and Kincardine (1811-1863), signed a treaty in Edo on August 26, 1858.

The first Japanese contacts with British medicine were through the reading of texts in English by Benjamin Hobson, M.R.C.S. (1816-1873),

---

[1] The Japanese subsequently signed similar treaties with the Netherlands, imperial Russia, and Britain.

[2] Thomas Rundall, ed., *Memorials of the Empire of Japon in the XVI and XVII Centuries* (London: Hakluyt Society, 1850), p. 169.

stationed in China for the London Missionary Society. These texts were compilations in Chinese drawn from English texts on anatomy and physiology, natural history and philosophy, surgery, medicine and materia medica, midwifery, and diseases of children.[3]

In August 1861, as the turbulence and tension mounted in Japan, Great Britain decided to add a surgeon to her legation. William Willis (M.D., Edinburgh), who was selected for the post, emerged from the agony and bloodshed of the decade that followed as a heroic and respected "Southern barbarian."

William Willis was born at Florence Court, County Fermanagh, northern Ireland, in 1837. In 1855 he enrolled at the Faculty of Medicine at the University of Glasgow, where he completed his premedical and preclinical studies.[4] He then transferred to the University of Edinburgh, the most prestigious medical faculty in Britain, and graduated in 1859. During his final years at the university, Willis earned a Membership in the Royal College of Surgeons, Edinburgh. Willis's graduation thesis was entitled "Theory of Ulceration."[5] The referees, from a faculty not noted for lavishing praise, were moved to comment on it, "Sensible Essay" and "Very Fair."

Edinburgh was a magnet for students from the British Empire, and its large classes restricted opportunities for practical bedside instruction. So it was that Willis took the "high road" to London, where he could walk the wards and gain practical skills in surgery and medicine at Middlesex Hospital. He now held a license from the London Society of Apothecaries.

He had been indoctrinated with the Edinburgh tradition that encouraged graduates in medicine and engineering to enter service in the colonies and the military. thus, after eighteen months at Middlesex spent primarily in surgery, he successfully applied for the newly established post of surgeon attached to the British embassy in Japan.

Standing well over six feet tall and large-boned, Willis must have made a dramatic initial impact in Japan. Not only did he tower over the Japanese but most of his countrymen as well. As a member of the embassy commented, "How he got into his little Japanese house and how, once in, he ever got out again remained as big a mystery as that of the apple in the dumpling."[6]

The respect with which other people regarded Willis is eloquently expressed by some comments of his closest friend, Ernest Satow (1843-1929), a diplomat and linguist who shared Willis's love for Japan. Satow stressed Willis's conscientiousness, his tenderness and sympathy toward

[3]K. Chi Min Wong and Lien-Teh Wu, *History of Chinese Medicine* (Tientsin: Tientsin Press, 1934), pp. 220-21.

[4]The information on Willis as a student is by courtesy of D. J. Cronin, senior administrative officer, Faculty of Medicine, University of Edinburgh.

[5]Information on Willis's doctoral thesis is by courtesy of the Keeper of Manuscripts, University Library, Edinburgh.

[6]Quoted in Pat Barr, *The Coming of the Barbarian. The Opening of Japan to the West, 1853-1879* (New York: E. P. Dutton, 1967), p. 154.

patients, his devotion to his profession, and his fearlessness in exposing himself to personal risks.[7]

Willis's professional career in Japan was intertwined with the turbulence that characterized the final decade of Tokugawa rule and its attendant hatred of foreigners, a situation of mutual animosity. Willis first personally encountered this attitude in September 1862. An unyielding tradition held that passersby meeting the retinue of a *daimyo* on the road must clear the thoroughfare, often turning their backs as an indication that they were not worthy to view such an august presence. In mid-September 1862, the *daimyo* of Satsuma and his retinue returning from Edo met a party of four British excursionists at Namamugi, near Kanagawa. This *daimyo* was the most antiforeign of the *tozama* lords. The British party did not pay sufficient obeisance and was brutally attacked by sword-swinging, outraged *samurai.* A woman in the group escaped with only her hat slashed, but the three men were wounded, one C. Lennox Richardson fatally. Willis, rushing to the scene from his post at Kanagawa, passed the samurai, who brandished swords "reeking with the blood of Englishmen."[8]

The ensuing five years were devoid of military medical activity for Willis, and he devoted his time to medical care of the foreign legations and to gaining fluency in Japanese. In 1864, as director of a makeshift smallpox hospital in Yokohama, he prevented an outbreak from becoming an epidemic.

The profound changes that were bringing about the decline and fall of the Tokugawa shogunate also carried Willis to the summit of his career as a military surgeon in Japan. On November 19, 1867, Tokugawa Keiki (also Yoshinobu) (1837-1913), the fifteenth shogun, abdicated, and the emperor, long sequestered in Miyako, became the actual ruler of Japan. He was Mutsuhito, a lad of fifteen years, but because of his youth actual power in the early years rested in the hands of the younger samurai of the *tozama* clans. These architects of the new Japan were military men at heart, but they recognized that the achievement of military might depended on a strong economic, intellectual, and social base. In order to establish these conditions, they embarked on a period of borrowing and adapting from Western culture that is unparalleled in modern history. As the new Japan began to take shape, a major question arose: "Which system of medicine should Japan adopt?" Willis became a central figure in the making of the decision.

Sir Rutherford Alcock, who served as British ambassador from December 21, 1858, to December 24, 1864, had encouraged the continuation of rule by the Tokugawa shogunate. However, Sir Harry Smith Parkes (1828-1885), who succeeded him on July 18, 1865, committed the British Empire to the restoration of the emperor. Parkes, a brilliant and outspoken man of fiery temperament, had spent twenty-four years in China and had

---

[7] Sir Ernest Satow, *A Diplomat in Japan* (London: Seeley Sons & Co., 1921), p. 31.
[8] Ibid., p. 52.

become well-versed in the ways of the Orient. As a high Japanese official commented, he was "the only foreigner in Japan whom we could not twist around our little finger."[9]

The year 1868 marked the last desperate efforts of the Tokugawa adherents to defeat the imperial forces, and the country was in a precarious state. The shogun moved to Osaka, and, as the rallying point for his followers, that city became a tinderbox. The major foreign diplomats sought the greater security of Hyogo (now Kobe), where their men-of-war rode at anchor.

That year began with Willis's promotion to the rank of vice-consul for the legation. His first adventure on the battlefield came when a crucial battle was fought on January 27 between Tokugawa forces advancing on Miyako and imperial troops from Satsuma and Choshu fiefs. They fought at Toba and Fushimi, two villages seven miles southeast of Kyoto, and the imperial troops suffered about 150 casualties. They lacked adequate surgical care, and Oyama Iwao (1842-1916), a military leader of Satsuma who had heard of Willis's surgical prowess, learned of his presence in Hyogo, some forty miles distant. Godai Tomoatsu (1837-1885), a Satsuma samurai, and Terajima Munenori (1832-1893), who had studied Dutch medicine, sought Parkes's approval for the use of Willis's services. Satow recalled: "The chief replied that the alleviation of suffering in the case of human being was always a pleasure."[10]

Willis and Satow with Oyama as military escort left Kobe for Kyoto by way of Osaka on the morning of February 16 aboard the gunboat H.M.S. *Cockchafer.* Heretofore, no foreigner had ever entered the imperial city, and Saigo requested the court to lift the ban. Willis and Satow were detained in Osaka because permission for the remainder of their trip had not come from the court. They were allowed to leave the city only after Willis threatened to abandon his mission and after Oyama volunteered to assure their safety. The official permits awaited them when they reached Fushimi at midnight—but now they met a new obstacle. A detachment of Satsuma samurai had been detailed to escort them through the lines, but when the warriors discovered that they were to protect foreigners, many of them refused. They were mollified, however, and at noon on February 18, 1868, Willis and Satow became the first foreigners to enter Kyoto.

The Satsuma and Choshu casualties had been carried to the Yogen-in, a building of the Sokoku-ji temple, just north of the imperial palace.[11] Among those whom Willis treated was Saigo Judo (also Tsugumichi), the younger brother of Saigo Takamori, and this act may have engendered the important friendship that developed between Willis and the older Saigo.

[9]James Murdoch, *A History of Japan,* vol. 3 (London: Kegan Paul, Trench, Trubner & Co., 1926), p. 757.

[10]Satow, *Diplomat in Japan,* p. 330.

[11]Shokoku-ji temple of the Rinzai sect was first erected in 1382. It adjoins the campus of Doshisha University, the first Christian university in Japan, founded in 1873 by Joseph Niijima. (See chapter 7.)

It was at Sokoku-ji that Willis performed the first major military surgery in Japan. The Japanese assigned to assist him were inexperienced, and Willis was obliged to carry out all procedures, including bandaging, by himself. He patiently instructed his assistants in the use of dressings and was impressed with the facility that they acquired.

Late in March 1868 Willis became involved in another bloody incident precipitated by Japanese xenophobia in Miyako. Parkes, accompanied by Willis and a British military escort, was riding to the imperial palace for his first audience with the emperor. They were quartered at Chion-in, the chief temple of the Jodo sect, and their route led them through narrow lanes bordered by houses and shops with overhanging eaves. It was in one of these streets that they were attacked by two Japanese slashing out with their long swords. The British lancers, hemmed in by the cramped lanes, could not elevate their shafts because of the eaves. Twelve of the party were wounded, and one of the Japanese was killed; Willis rendered first aid and continued to care for them after they had been carried back to Chion-in. Deeply embarrassed by this incident, the imperial court sent a legation to apologize to Parkes, but he insisted on having a written apology and a public proclamation attesting that the emperor was sincerely committed to developing friendly relations with foreign powers. When the emperor met his demands, Parkes proceeded without incident to the palace for an audience.

On March 31 Willis returned to Yokohama with Parkes and the other members of the legation staff. He was destined to have only a brief respite from the battlefield, for on July 4 fighting broke out at Ueno in Edo. Willis established an emergency dressing station in Tozenji temple, which was serving as the temporary home of the British legation when he arrived in 1861. Once again the condition of the casualties was deplorable, since the treatment of their wounds had been amateurish at best. Willis worked round-the-clock for several weeks; as the patient load grew, he took over a converted barracks and a tea warehouse.

Since Willis's official duties as vice-consul required his presence at the legation in Yokohama, he asked that the casualties be transferred there. At first, a large residence proved sufficient, but as the number of patients increased daily, nearby brothels and a former military barracks were brought into service. Willis soon found that he could not simultaneously fulfill his duties as vice-consul and military surgeon. Joseph Bower Siddall (M.D., Aberdeen), who had just arrived to succeed Willis as medical officer at the legation, assumed the day-to-day responsibilities for the wounded.

Siddall submitted to the foreign office a report on his work as a military surgeon from June 15, 1868, to March 1, 1869.[12] Under his tutelage, the Japanese surgeons soon became adept at bandaging and splinting.

---

[12] J. B. Siddall, "Surgical experiences in military hospitals in Japan," St. Thomas's Hospital Reports, London, n.s., 1874, 5: 85-112.

They learned surgical techniques by practicing on extremities that Siddall had just amputated. Because of Willis's successful amputations at Kyoto, some of the patients assumed that this was the only form of treatment for a fracture.

In mid-November, Parkes agreed to a request by the new government that Siddall be sent to Edo to take charge of another temporary military hospital in the abandoned Todo *yashiki*.[13] The hall-like rooms in the main residence were admirably suited to serve as wards, but the patients preferred to have individual rooms, even though these were quite small. After a lifetime of sleeping on six-by-three-foot *tatami* (mats), the patients found the hospital bed a new experience. They ignored sanitary practice and fouled the beds with liquids, dirt, and excrement. It was only after Siddall had ripped to pieces in their presence several stinking mattresses that the patients began to observe hygienic practices.

The sanitary conditions on the grounds were as deplorable as those in the wards. As in most *yashiki,* drainage was minimal, and the frequent rains left the place a quagmire. The problems of filth were compounded by the failure of attendants to collect refuse routinely; when they did so, they tossed it into poorly covered ditches beside the hospital. In frustration, Siddall refused to enter the hospital until the ditches were cleared and the laborers systematically collected all refuse on a daily schedule. Siddall continued to have problems with sporadic cases of gangrene, which he attributed to the muck.

A nurse was considered to be at about the same social level as a prostitute and came from a similarly humble background. These factors, combined with the inferior, obedient role of women, made the nurses totally lacking in the firmness so characteristic of British nurses. On at least one occasion, for example, Siddall found it necessary to bathe a young patient himself, because the lad had intimidated the nurses when they had tried to do so. Since it was a military hospital, nurses were plentiful. In general, Siddall was approving and praised their sympathy with patients: "These women, as a rule, seemed to perform their duties very well, and I have seen them weep bitterly on the fatal termination of a case."[14]

Under Siddall's direction, drugs from Holland and Britain replaced the Chinese materia medica. Prescriptions were compounded by practitioners who in many instances had only a smattering of instruction in pharmaceutical procedures. Serious blunders often occurred, especially with the more complicated European compounds, and Siddall soon found it necessary to supervise personally the preparation of all drug mixtures.

The administration of medications also was fraught with difficulties. An eggnog mixture for convalescent patients often became the excuse for a communal drinking session: "I have seen half a dozen friends sitting talking to a wounded man [commented Siddall], and all drinking brandy-and-egg mixture with the greatest relish."[15]

The Japanese lived by the sword, and one patient told Siddall that he "did not like this fighting at a distance, for you fought as it were in the dark, but when you fought with swords it was so nice to kill your enemy and see what you had done."[16] Siddall attributed the paucity of sword wounds to the very fact that the man who fell with such a wound was killed immediately by his enemy. The wounds Siddall treated were inflicted exclusively by rifles and muskets—from every variety of breech loader to an ordinary smoothbore.

The patience and fortitude of the Japanese casualties were admirable. They seemed deficient, though, in what Siddall called "nerve power." This made them more susceptible to postoperative shock and may have accounted for the unexpected death of several patients in the immediate postoperative period. After several months of handling battlefield casualties, both Willis and Siddall came to the conclusion that conservative management was preferable to amputation, with its attendant high mortality.[17]

When the imperial forces moved north in the autumn of 1868, Willis again served as their surgeon. He left Edo in October on a painful two-month journey of 600 miles, on foot or cramped in a shoe-box-like *norimono* (palanquin). The trek was largely across windswept, mountainous terrain. At Takata, Willis once again collided with the hatred of foreigners. While he was passing a guard house, he was rushed by the guards, who tried to force him to bow. Willis broke away, refusing to comply, and demanded an apology from the chief of the guards, which the latter declined to give. Willis would not pass the barrier and sent a letter to the *daimyo* demanding redress. Soon, two representatives of the *daimyo* arrived with profuse apologies. The chief guard was required to make a formal apology; he also made the traditional offer to commit *seppuku* (suicide by slashing the belly), but Willis in turn declined the honor.[18]

The site of the battle between the imperial and the Tokugawa forces was Aizu, a clan city with an almost impregnable fortress-castle at Wakamatsu. The Aizu, with roots going back to the third shogun, Tokugawa Iemitsu, and the Sendai clans were the last clans to fight for the Tokugawa. Fierce fighting raged for a month before the Wakamatsu citadel was captured on October 29 by the imperial forces.

Upon his arrival, Willis found that the casualties of the imperial army were being cared for adequately. On the other hand, the Aizu "were in a

[15] Ibid., p. 81.

[16] Ibid., p. 111.

[17] Ibid., p. 107. Siddall managed 114 cases with compound comminuted fractures of the extremities. The mortality from amputations was 60 percent, while for cases treated conservatively it was only 20 percent.

[18] Great Britain, *Sessional Papers* (Commons), vol. 64 (1869), pp. 33-38.

deplorable state of filth and wretchedness, and excepting a ration of rice, nothing else was allowed them." He persuaded the authorities at Wakamatsu to supply their wounded with food and regular sugical and medical care. Willis personally cared for 600 men and supervised the care of some 1,000 others on both sides. He performed only thirty-eight amputations, ranging from the removal of a finger to a complex hip-joint amputation. Of these patients, half survived.

In a memorandum on his expedition, Willis commented on the cruelty exhibited by the imperial forces: "I had occasion frequently to observe the significant absence of wounded prisoners and as often as opportunity presented I pointed out the inhumanity of a wanton sacrifice of life." Their excuse was that the Aizu troops had "reviled and insulted the Mikado's authority so effusively that it was found impossible to spare even the lives of the wounded."[19]

Matsumoto Ryojun (1832-1907), surgeon general of the Tokugawa armed forces—who, as will be recalled, was Pompe van Meerdevoort's deputy at Nagasaki—was among the prisoners captured at Wakamatsu. Soon after Pompe returned to Holland, Matsumoto re-joined the shogunate as chief physician and vice-director of *Seiyo Igakujo,* under Otsuki Shunsai, a *hatamoto* ("flag person," used for samurai who served the shogun directly) physician. Ogata Koan succeeded Otsuki in 1862 but died the following year, and Matsumoto became director. He was designated surgeon general of the Tokugawa armed forces when the hostilities with the imperial army erupted.

Together with the remaining forces of the Tokugawa, Matsumoto retreated to Wakamatsu in April 1868 and was caring for casualties in the field when he was taken prisoner. After twenty months he was released and opened a medical school, Ranchusha, with a hospital, Ranchu-in, at Waseda in Tokyo. In May 1871, Matsumoto accepted an invitation from his former enemies to organize a division of military medicine for the imperial army. When the military establishment was reorganized in the spring of 1873, he was appointed to the post of surgeon general to the imperial forces, the same position he had formerly held with their enemy. He retired from service in 1885, was created a peer, then a baron, and died in 1907.

In 1858 a group of physicians trained in Western medicine founded Shutojo (vaccination institute). These founders were Ito Genboku, Totsuka Seikai, Otsuki Shunsai, Hayashi Dokai, Mitsukuri Gempo, Takeuchi Gendo, and Miyake Ryosai.[20] They were joined by seventy-seven other physicians; the shogunate granted sponsorship, and Kawaji Toshiaki, the *Kanjo-bugyo* (a *Bakufu* financial official), donated a piece of property at

[19]Ibid., enclosure 1 in no. 7, p. 35.

[20]Willis Norton Whitney, "Notes on the history of medical progress in Japan," *Transactions of the Asiatic Society of Japan,* vol. 12 (Yokohama: R. Meiklenohn & Co., 1885), p. 343.

Otamagaike, Kanda. Fire destroyed the first building in 1858, but the following year a new structure was erected at Shitaya, Izumibashi-dori. When the shogunate assumed control and responsibility for financial support two years later, limited instruction in Western medicine—anatomy, chemistry, and materia medica—was inaugurated and dormitories were erected. Otsuki Shunsai, a *hatamoto* physician, was appointed superintendent. Upon his death in 1862, Ogata Koan was summoned from Osaka to become director. One year after assuming the directorship Ogata Koan died; it was then that Matsumoto Ryojun became the director.

The Meiji government took over the school on June 18, 1868, and changed its name to Igakujo. Hayashi Dokai (also Kenkai), who had accompanied Pompe van Meerdervoort in 1862, was appointed director.

In December 1868, Willis returned to Edo and for his heroism became the first foreigner and commoner to receive seven imperial brocades from the emperor. The British foreign secretary, George Villiers, fourth earl of Clarendon, issued an official commendation.

The Meiji government took steps to convert Siddall's military hospital to a general hospital at the Todo *yashiki* and to expand instruction in Western medicine. Parkes and Satow pressed for Willis to be appointed director of the institution. They knew that the Japanese were about to select a European system of medicine, and if Willis became director, the balance might well be tipped in Britain's favor.

With this objective in mind, Satow visited the hospital on January 10 and discussed strategy with Siddall and Willis. The plan they evolved was to tell Siddall's Japanese associate, Ishigami Ryosaku (a practitioner from Satsuma who worked at the hospital and was married to Ine Siebold, daughter of Philipp von Siebold), that Siddall was about to be recalled to the British legation. Ishigami was to advise the court that the hospital urgently needed Willis as its chief. Their strategy succeeded: Willis was appointed director and chief surgeon and Siddall returned to a full-time post at the legation.

The Japanese staff at Igakujo was headed by Maeda Shinsuke of Kagoshima as dean; in a few months, he was succeeded by Ogata Koreyoshi (also Ijun). Tsuboi Ishun (also Hoshu), Tashiro Kazunori, and Ishigami Ryosaku served as assistant teachers.

The realities of the situation, including the ban on dissection and the absence of teaching laboratories, limited Willis's teaching program to materia medica, surgery, and internal medicine. The *Nikko Kibum* ("Japanese lecture record") of Shimamura Teiho, one of the students, includes notes from his lectures on internal medicine and surgery. He discussed the physiology, pathology, and treatment of gastritis, causes of dyspepsia, and stenosis of the esophagus. Demonstrations illustrated the technique for tracheotomy under chloroform anesthesia in children with diphtheria. For aphonia and chronic inflammation of the throat, Willis recommended caustic silver, and for dyspnoea, swabbing with mercuric chloride. His most enduring contribution during the ten months he served as director was the introduction of teaching at the bedside.

A year after he returned to the legation, Siddall became responsible for a signal advance in public health—compulsory smallpox vaccination. After Mohnike introduced vaccination, the *Bakufu* had been unwilling to endorse it officially, because such an action would imply the approval of a foreign technique. The new Meiji government had what it considered more pressing problems until in the winter of 1870-71, a severe epidemic of smallpox swept Tokyo; Siddall and Dr. George Newton, a British naval surgeon, launched a campaign to persuade the new government to establish a vaccination program. Newton volunteered to develop and supervise free vaccination centers for nationals of all nations as well as smallpox hospitals. (He also organized the first venereal disease hospitals in Japanese ports between 1867 and his death in 1871.) The plan was warmly embraced at a meeting of all British and American medical men in the Tokyo-Yokohama area and by Sir Harry Parkes. The government representative at the meeting, Iseki Sayemon, pledged that every effort would be made to carry out the plan.

On March 15, 1871, Shutokan (vaccination office) opened at Toko (East College), the new name for Igakujo. Shutokan became the head-quarters of a network that combined free vaccination with the training of vaccinators: "the first statutory preventive rules against epidemics in Japan."[21] Siddall and Newton's goal was achieved in 1874, when the government made vaccination compulsory. Two years later, the regulation was tightened to require vaccination during the first year of life, and on two subsequent occasions at intervals of five to seven years.

For his accomplishments in military surgery and his leadership in introducing vaccination, Siddall became the first foreigner to receive the Order of the Rising Sun.[22] Siddall returned to England and practiced medicine on Ross-on-Wye until the age of fifty. He died at Great Malvern, England, on July 4, 1925, at the age of eighty-five.

The fifth article of the Charter Oath of Five Articles, proclaimed in the spring of 1868, stated: "Wisdom and knowledge shall be sought all over the world to establish firmly the foundations of the empire." Missions visited America and Western Europe to determine which systems were most suitable for Japan. Foreign advisors were invited to introduce modernization in a variety of fields. Railways, postal systems, and harbors followed British models. The Dutch provided the first naval vessels and instructors but

[21] F. Ohtani, *One Hundred Years of Health Progress in Japan* (Tokyo: Taihei Printing Co., 1971), p. 28.

[22] The heraldry of feudal Japan had not included knighthoods or other forms of recognition for distinguished services. Six orders were established in 1875, and the Order of the Rising Sun became the decoration most frequently bestowed upon foreigners for meritorious services.

were later supplanted in these areas by Britain and America. The French pattern served for the new army until after the Franco-Prussian War the German model superseded it. The legal code was Napoleonic, as was the concept of a highly centralized governmental structure. Education, agriculture, and the opening of Hokkaido to development drew on American influence and experts.

Prussian nationalism, political philosophy, and bureaucratic structure soon became the basis of the Japanese national organization. Ito Hirobumi (1841-1909), who supervised the drafting of the new constitution, followed the directives of the "Iron Chancellor," Otto von Bismarck (1815-1898), Europe's most powerful statesman. Bismarck told him to shun democracy altogether: Japan must adopt imperial rule with a tightly controlled elected assembly, responsible solely to the emperor and not to the people.

In March 1868 the government announced that a system of Western medicine would be adopted. The choice would be between the German and the English approaches. In December of that year an ordinance was promulgated that established the requirement of an examination to practice medicine: all active physicians, including those who practiced *Kampo,* were required to pass the examination.

At that time, German medicine had become preeminent in the Western world. Wilhelm von Humboldt (1767-1835), the chief architect of the new German educational system, believed that medical faculties should be rooted in universities and that an indissoluble bond linked investigation and teaching. Thus, modern biomedical research had its first flowering in the German universities, beginning with the physiology laboratory of Johannes E. Purkinje (1787-1869) at Breslau in 1824 and the first university-based chemistry institute, established by Justus von Liebig (1803-1873) at Giessen in 1826. Research was emphasized to the same degree by professors in the clinical as in the basic-science departments.

The burst of national pride and creative energy that exploded in Germany after her victories in the Seven Weeks' War of 1866 gave the universities scientific laboratories to match the talent and creative vigor of their professors. As Louis Pasteur mourned in 1868 from his attic laboratories, "Rich and large laboratories have been growing in Germany for the last thirty years and many more are still being built; at Berlin and at Bonn two palaces, worth four million francs each, are being erected for chemical studies."[23] On the other hand, English medical schools in the nineteenth century were hospital based. The basic sciences were neglected in favor of practical clinical instruction at the bedside.

Apart from Germany's position of world leadership in medicine, factors in Japanese medical history placed Germany in a favored position. As we have noted earlier, German physicians had been preeminent in Tokugawa

[23] R. Vallery-Radot, *The Life of Pasteur,* trans. R. L. Devonshire (New York: Doubleday, Page & Co., 1927), p. 152.

Japan: Engelbert Kaempfer, the scientific discoverer of the empire; Philipp Franz Balthasar von Siebold; and Otto Mohnike. The prevalence of German medical texts had also elevated the status of German medicine.

In 1869, the government solicited the opinion of two physicians, Sagara Chian (also Tomoyasu) (1836-1906) and Iwasa Jun (1835-1912), on the system of medicine that should be adopted. Sagara was of a samurai family of the Saga fief, whose *daimyo* was the famed Nabeshima Naomasa (also Kanso), who put forward Okuma Shigenobu, Soejima Taneomi, and several other leaders of the restoration. Sagara had studied medicine at Nagasaki with Bauduin and in 1868 was summoned to Tokyo to serve as chief of medical schools, to encourage the development of new schools, and to separate the *Bakufu* schools from the new institutions. Iwasa Jun, of a samurai family in Echizen fief, had also studied Western medicine at Nagasaki.

Sagara and Iwasa favored German medicine but were sensitive to the prestige of Willis and of British medicine. They sought the advice of Reverend Guido Fridolin Verbeck (1830-1898), a Dutch Reformed missionary from America who, as their former teacher at Nagasaki, had become a chief counselor to the builders of the New Japan. He told them that German medicine had to be their choice. At the end of 1869 the two Japanese submitted their recommendations that teachers of medicine should be invited from Germany.

Born in 1830 in Zeist, the Netherlands, Verbeck was baptized in the Moravian faith and after attending a sectarian preparatory school graduated in civil engineering from the polytechnic school at Utrecht. In response to an invitation from his brother-in-law, the Reverend George van Deurs, Verbeck immigrated to Green Bay, Wisconsin, in 1852. During a trip through Arkansas, he developed cholera and made a solemn vow that, if restored to health, he would consecrate his life to missionary service. Verbeck may also have been influenced by the long and rich tradition of the Moravian *Unitas Fratrum,* which sent missions to the most remote and difficult regions.[24] Verbeck fulfilled his vow by enrolling at the Dutch Reformed Theological Seminary, Auburn, New York, where he was licensed and ordained. He then answered an appeal for a Reformed missionary to go to Japan, and the long history of native Dutch practitioners serving at Nagasaki made him the sponsors' logical choice.[25]

[24] K. S. Latourette, *A History of Christian Missions in China* (London: Society for Promoting Christian Knowledge, 1929), p. 255.

[25] In 1855, a decision to send American missionaries to Japan had originated on the deck of the battleship *Minnesota* as she lay at anchor in Nagasaki Bay. S. Wells Williams, L.L.D. (1812-1884), the distinguished sinologist who had served as Perry's interpreter, discussed the newly opened mission field in Japan with the Reverend E. W. Syle and the ship's chaplain, the Reverend Henry Wood. They decided to send appeals for missionaries to the Dutch Reformed, Episcopal, and Presbyterian mission boards; the boards responded affirmatively. Verbeck was sponsored by the South Reformed Church, Fifth Avenue and Twenty-first Street, New York City.

Together with his new bride, Maria Manion Verbeck (1840-1911), whom he had converted to the Reformed faith while he was a theological student, the Reverend S. T. Brown, D.D., and a medical missionary, Duane B. Simmons, M.D., Verbeck arrived in Shanghai on the S.S. *Surprise,* on October 17, 1859. After discussing problems and opportunities in the Orient with Williams, the three missionaries sailed into Nagasaki Bay on November 7, 1859.

Two centuries of harsh interdicts against Christianity had left their mark, and Verbeck found the Japanese "not at all accessible touching religious matters. When the subject was mooted in the presence of a Japanese, his hand would almost involuntarily be applied to his throat, to indicate the extreme perilousness of such a topic."[26] As a further example, he cited the reaction of the governor of Hyogo prefecture, who, when asked if a local book agent could sell the English Bible, replied that if the man did so he would be sent immediately to prison.

Verbeck circumvented the ban against Christianity by using the New Testament as the text for his classes in English. (The Constitution of the United States served as a secondary text.) His students came from Nagasaki and the feudatories of southwest Japan, principally Satsuma and Choshu. On January 26, 1860, the Verbecks became the parents of the first Christian infant born in Japan.[27] They named their daughter Emma and gave her the middle name "Japonica" in honor of their new homeland.

The life of a foreigner in Nagasaki was perilous, and in 1863 Verbeck and his family moved behind the palisades of Dejima for safety. They spent the summer of that year at Shanghai, where Verbeck studied Chinese in order to read the more scholarly Japanese books.

After their return to Nagasaki in November of 1863, Verbeck was informed that because of the attainments of two of his first students, the governor of Nagasaki had proposed him to the *Bakufu* for a high educational position. Verbeck would become the principal of a new governmental school, to teach foreign language and science. The request was endorsed, and Verbeck's school soon attracted the best young minds from the *tozama* fiefs. They included Iwakura Tomomi (1825-1883), who as a senior minister of the Meiji government would lead the mission to America and Europe in 1871-1873; Okuma Shigenobu (1838-1922), who would also become a senior minister; and Soejima Taneomi (1828-1905), who would succeed Iwakura at the foreign ministry in 1870 and later serve as envoy to Peking.

In 1869 Komatsu Tatewaki (1835-1870), another former student and now vice-minister of foreign affairs, told Verbeck that the government wished him to come to Tokyo and strengthen the teaching of foreign languages at Kaiseisho (enlightenment school). As with many other develop-

---

[26]G. F. Verbeck, "Early mission days in Japan," *The Japan Advertiser* (Tokyo, 30 October 1926).

[27]W. E. Griffis, *Verbeck of Japan, a Citizen of No Country: A Life Story of Foundation Work Inaugurated by Guido Fridolin Verbeck* (New York: Revell Co., 1900), p. 90.

ments, its establishment had been precipitated by the arrival of Commodore Perry in 1853. After his departure the shogunate solicited advice from leading *daimyo* and scholars as to Western learning. Katsu Rintaro (1823-1899), an advisor to the *Bakufu,* recommended a full-scale adoption of Western studies:

A school for instruction and training should be established. . . . For its library there should be collected all sorts of books in Japanese, Chinese, and Dutch having to do with military matters and gunnery, and . . . in the school orders should be given to establish faculties for the study of astronomy, geography, science, military science, gunner, fortifications, and mechanics.[28]

Katsu's proposal was accepted in 1854, although more conservative minds preferred a more traditional program in order to limit the influence of Western techniques and philosophy.

The original name assigned to the school was Yogakusho (institute for Western learning), but after one year it was changed to Bansho Shirabesho (institute for the investigation of barbarian books). At the beginning, the school emphasized teaching in Dutch, but owing to the ascendancy of other Western powers, German, French, and English texts were added.[29] The men connected with the institution were former samurai, some of whom became influential members of the Meiji bureaucracy.

At the time of Verbeck's death in 1898, his crucial role in the decision for German medicine was attested to by Surgeon General Ishiguro Tadanori:

Drs. Iwasa, Sagara, Hasegawa Yasushi, and I held the view that the science of medicine should be German. How we were ridiculed and criticized by the public! Dr. Verbeck was already in those times respected and believed in by the people. One day Dr. Sagara got an interview with him and talked about the necessity of enforcing their opinion about the science of medicine. The American teacher expressed his sympathy with our view. It was through his advice to the government that German professors of the science came to be employed. The present prosperity of the science owes a great deal to the deceased doctor.[30]

Following the decision to adopt German medicine, the embarrassing question arose as to how to compensate William Willis for his services to

---

[28]Quoted in Numata Jiro, *Bakumatsu Yogakushi* (Tokyo: Tokoshoin, 1950), pp. 56-57.

[29]"As this happened the nature of *Bansho Shirabesho* began to change, and in 1863 in response to a memorial from the director, its name was changed to *Kaiseijo*. It now offered instruction in Dutch, English, French, German, and Russian as well as a variety of useful arts" (M. B. Jansen, "New materials for the intellectual history of nineteenth-century Japan," *Harvard Journal of Asiatic Studies,* 1957, *20,* nos. 3 and 4: 582. Oddly enough, when Jansen studied the collection of foreign books from the *Bansho Shirabesho* in the 1950s, he found only a single medical text. He attributed this absence of medical books to the popularity of medicine and the public zeal for books relating to it.

[30]Quoted in Griffis, *Verbeck of Japan,* p. 211.

the country. Sagara Chian requested Willis's old friend Saigo Takamori to invite the Scot to develop Western medicine in distant Kagoshima. Willis was eager to stay in Japan and assented, insisting on a four-year contract for the reason that it would be impossible to establish Western medicine in two years. *Gaimusho* (foreign ministry) approved his terms on December 3, 1869, and at the end of the year Willis left for Kagoshima accompanied by Hayashi Bokuan, his pupil and assistant at Daibyoin.

Prior to Willis's arrival at Kagoshima the *daimyo,* Shimazu, had established a school that combined *Kampo* and Western medicine. It was later separated into two schools, and Willis assumed leadership of the Igakujo, which was moved to Jokoji temple. A *han* hospital, Akakura-Byoin ("red go-down hospital"), of Western design and red brick construction, was erected at Ogawa-cho, near the medical school. When the prefectural system was introduced in 1869, the medical school and hospital became the responsibility of the prefectural government.

Willis established a four-year medical course that included instruction in English and world geography as well as anatomy, physiology, pathology, internal medicine, surgery, ophthalmology, pediatrics, and obstetrics. He lectured in English with Takagi Kanehiro and Mitamura Hajime as interpreters, and the lectures were later transcribed and distributed to the students. Willis found only a handful of medical books, but through purchases in Tokyo and other acquisitions, he developed an adequate stock of Western texts on internal medicine, midwifery and gynecology, pediatrics, and infectious diseases. In the Edinburgh tradition, he placed special emphasis on anatomy. As at Tokyo, he introduced the students to the practice of teaching at the bedside.

Willis also offered a two-year course on *chozai* (the preparation of medications). Upon completion of the course, students returned to the villages as *Ranpoi* (Dutch-system doctors), to serve as dispensers.

Willis stated his views on medical education in May 1871 in a letter to Oyama Tsunayoshi, the *kenrei* (governor) of Satsuma. He stressed the importance of combining the lectures with practical instruction and the necessity of a teaching hospital to make this effective.[31] A total of five to six hundred students from prefectures as distant as Aizu, Shizuoka, and Wakayama were attracted to Igakujo by Willis's renown. A significant number came with the sole objective of learning English.

Dental surgery was another area in which Willis was skillful, but he was limited by having at his disposal only instruments of ivory, wood, or tortoise shell. It was impossible to sterilize them satisfactorily, and he encountered continuing problems with infection.

Besides being a surgeon of acknowledged skill, Willis was a first-rate generalist. He taught the care and treatment of problems in internal medicine, female diseases, and disorders of the nose, throat, and eye. He is said to have performed the first iridectomy for glaucoma in Japan.

[31] Willis, Letter, March 1875.

Dr. Sato Hachiro, dean emeritus of Kagoshima University Faculty of Medicine, gives a lively account of Willis in the surgical theater:

He was very broadminded and liked *sake*. Before operations he tilted a big cup of wine and yet was dexterous in handling the knife. At the same time he was meticulous in his care of patients and especially with the use of chloroform—he counted the pulse and warned if it was too fast or too slow.[32]

And Willis could not tolerate sloppiness: "Often if his assistants made a mistake he scolded them severely, so they were all afraid of him."[33]

Willis was probably the first physician to open a free clinic solely for the sick poor in Japan. He was also a pioneer in the introduction of the following Western health practices in Japan: (1) vaccination against smallpox; (2) routine prepartum care of pregnant women; (3) precautions against the consumption of contaminated meat; (4) prevention of syphilis; and (5) the establishment of European sanitary and hygienic standards for the hospital. Despite his arduous schedule, he was always available for house calls, of which he made several each day.

The Emperor Meiji visited Kagoshima in 1872 and paid a special call at Akakura Byoin, in part to grant Willis a *tenran* ("Observe the heavenly"), or audience. The emperor observed the work of the students. In a traditional gesture of goodwill, he left a gift of money (*shukoryo*) for the purchase of food and beverages for the patients.

At the end of May 1874, Willis joined a military expedition to Formosa in order to chastise the Chinese. Satsuma considered the Ryukyu Islands part of its domain, and aborigines in Formosa, which was considered a part of China, had murdered fifty-four Ryukyu fishermen. China refused to assume responsibility for the incident, and Saigo Takamori insisted on the expedition of invasion. Japanese officials regarded the situation as an opportunity to flex their military "muscles," and Japan's armed services were eager for a fight. With a force of 3,600 soldiers and 289 sailors, the Japanese gained a clean-cut military victory and, of far greater importance, a ringing diplomatic victory over China. By recognizing Japan's legal right to protect her subjects, China gave her a legal claim to the Ryukyu Islands, and five years later they officially became part of the Japanese empire.

Malaria proved to be the major health problem of the expedition, and the most serious cases were admitted to the Nagasaki teaching hospital. Willis himself contracted malaria, and it contributed to a subsequent deterioration of his health.

Among Willis's patients were a Kagoshima samurai, Enatsu Juro, and his pretty daughter, Yaeko. She was a devout Christian and a student of

[32] Hachiro Sato, *Eii "William Willis" Ryakuden* (Kagoshima-Ken Kyoin Gojokai Insatsubu, 1968), p. 54.
[33] Ibid.

waka, a form of Japanese poetry. Willis wished to marry her and was required to submit to the Japanese tradition of a *nakodo* (go-between) in order to make the formal proposal and plans for the union. The marriage took place in 1871; their only child, Albert Willis, was born in 1873 at their home in Kajiya-machi.

Willis's four-year contract expired in 1875, and he returned to England on March 1 of that year. His achievements were noteworthy: the hospital and medical school were firmly established, the number of students had increased steadily, and the graduates included representatives of the leading families.

At the time of his departure, Willis presented a detailed report to Oyama Tsunayoshi on his stewardship at Kagoshima:

First of all I am contented that my efforts in the instruction of European medicine have been rewarded by success and that local people have come to confide in me because this type of medical treatment has been proved to be remarkably effective.

I have taught my students by giving them lectures on one day followed by medical practices on the next day. This has proved beneficial to both medical students and patients.

Up to this date more than fifteen thousand patients have visited our hospital and in addition to them we have given medical treatment to several thousand of go-and-see patients at their homes. Diseases ranged from ordinary ones to serious illnesses. Operations have also been performed at our hospital covering incisions, amputations of thighs, and others.

You will come to know the above facts by observing the many patients in our hospital and the one hundred and fifty medical students, some of them coming from the other prefectures and isolated islands to attend our Medical School. I also would like to inform you that a certain prefecture in an attempt to establish a similar hospital to ours has asked us for several medical staff members and that no small number of alumni have been appointed to positions of high-ranking medical officers in the Japanese navy.

Willis went on to discuss the improvement of hygiene and public health:

As to sanitary conditions in Kagoshima I am contented to know that many reforms and improvements have been accomplished in the past five years. Taking an example, raw beef previously served among local people has been discontinued.

Although remarkable reforms have been made with local hygiene there still are several problems left untouched. The most important problem to be solved as early as possible is the construction of water works and sewerage facilities to keep the city clean and sanitary. In addition, let me point out that in every medical field, prevention is more important than treatment of diseases.

From European countries I intend to obtain the knowledge and technology necessary for the best and most economical construction of waterworks and sewerage in Kagoshima. On my revisiting Japan, you will be kept informed of the progress. I also shall make every effort to give the most effective medical treatment to patients of leprosy often observed in Japan. When I learned that my fellow doctors, medical students, and very many patients were looking forward to my early return to Kagoshima I was convinced that what I had done in Kagoshima was beneficial to local communities.[34]

Willis returned to Kagoshima on April 29, 1876, and signed a new contract for three years.

Willis's second tour at Kagoshima was cut short by the Seinan (west-south) War, precipitated by Saigo Takamori. Saigo had been the senior member of a small group of samurai who were active in the restoration movement. Saigo became the supreme military leader of the armed forces, but as a "country boy" who clung to the bucolic life, he soon professed disgust with the extravagant life-style of his colleagues. Their successive moves to strip the samurai class of its exclusive status further disturbed him. The decisive incident came in 1873, with the deterioration of relations with Korea. Thoroughly disillusioned, Saigo returned to Satsuma. He continued his friendship with Willis and encouraged the development of Igakujo and Akakura-Byoin.

The first of a series of risings by a group of frustrated ex-samurai occurred in 1874, in Saga prefecture of northern Kyushu. Others followed, and suspicious eyes turned to Saigo Takamori as the fomenter of the revolts. The risings reached a climax in January 1877, when Saigo and his followers launched the Seinan War (also known as the Satsuma Rebellion).

Two totally contradictory opinions are held about Willis and his relationship to the Seinan War. We do know that Saigo came to Willis's home to discuss his determination to lead the rebellion. The generally accepted view is that Willis rejected outright the idea of the war. An opposing view is that Willis volunteered to join Saigo as medical officer, but that Saigo, who was obsessed with the idea of his own death, refused the offer because he believed that if he died he would be unable to protect Willis.

The question arose again on August 16, 1908, in an article in *Kagoshima Shimbun:* "Willis wished to treat the wounded soldiers, both friend and foe. But he was foreigner, and if Saigo had been defeated, Willis would have been an enemy of the emperor and there would have been serious problems."

At the outbreak of the Seinan War, Sir Harry Parkes, recalling Willis's friendship with Saigo, sent a man-of-war to Kagoshima to bring him to Tokyo; Willis came aboard with Yaeko and their son, Albert. The deck officer told Willis that since this was a vessel of the Queen's Navy, they could not permit a woman on board. Willis retorted that this was his family, it was an emergency, and he could not abandon them. Finally, they

---

[34]Hachiro Sato, *Dr. William Willis (1837-1894)—A Great Contributor to Western Medicine in Japan* (Kagoshima Prefectural Teachers Association Printing Section, 1968), pp. 5-8.

agreed to take Willis and his family to Nagasaki, whence they sailed to Tokyo.

When the fighting ended in September 1877, Willis returned to Kagoshima with his family. He was flattered to learn that the leading surgeons of the rebel forces were former students of his and that their skillful care of casualties had impressed the medical officers of the imperial army. Since Akakura-Byoin and Igakujo had been damaged and stripped, Willis had to renew his programs in teaching and patient care with only limited resources at his disposal.

When his three-year contract expired in the spring of 1881, Willis returned to Monmouth, where he practiced in partnership with his brother George. Albert accompanied him, while Yaeko remained in Kagoshima. At the same time, he continued to pursue his studies and earned diplomas as Member, Royal College of Physicians (London), and Fellow, Royal College of Surgeons (Edinburgh). In the meantime he enrolled Albert in a private school in London, but there was little contact between father and son.

In 1885 Willis's old friend Ernest Satow was named Her Majesty's Minister to the Kingdom of Siam, and he urged Willis to join him as medical officer. Willis's affection for the Orient was rekindled, and in 1885 he assumed responsibilities at Bangkok.

Siam presented a distressing example of a country primitive in medicine and health, since the drive for social reform initiated by King Rama IV (1851-1868) had not spread to the control of disease. There were only a few educated physicians, mostly missionaries concentrated in Bangkok. Medical care rested in the hands of Siamese and Chinese practitioners of traditional medicine, including a large number of Buddhist priests and outright quacks, who were known as *Moh* and *Maw Muangh*. Therapeutic practices consisted of incantations, herbs, and jealously guarded secret formulas handed down from father to son. A very popular and expensive medication, ground shark's tooth, was prescribed for practically all ailments. No regulations existed governing the practice of medicine, and any person could call himself a practitioner.

Public-health programs were totally lacking. Cholera and smallpox were the chief causes of the shockingly high death rate. Other communicable diseases included hookworm, malaria, and typhoid fever. Addiction to hashish was a major factor in the prevalence of insanity.

Three years after Willis's arrival, on the recommendation of H.R.H. Prince Damrong, who had studied in Europe, a royal medical college was established in an abandoned palace. The educational program focussed on surgery, medicine, and midwifery; there was also an abbreviated program to train native practitioners in indigenous medical practices.

Willis developed a large private practice that included King Rama V and his brother, Devawongze. Through this close relationship with the royal family, Willis was able to persuade the king to undertake major sanitary and moral reforms, including the abolition of concubinage and the improvement of prison conditions.

Two decades of stress in Japan and the enervating, unhealthy climate of Siam, exacerbated by an acute illness in 1892, forced Willis to return to England. There he divided his time between practice in Monmouth and participation in the medical sodalities in London. His passion for earning higher degrees was as strong as ever, and in 1893 he was awarded the Diploma of Public Health at Cambridge.

Willis joined his brother George at their family home in Ireland for the Christmas season in 1893. He succumbed to "bilious fever" and died on February 14.[35]

[35] *British Medical Journal,* 1894, *i:* 441.

5

German Medicine

The faculty of Medicine at the University of Berlin was the well-spring of modern medicine in Japan. Berlin served as the principal training ground for postgraduate study by the Japanese, who returned to Tokyo imbued with the spirit of German "philosophy" and the Prussian system of medical education. The influence of Berlin permeated the other imperial-university medical faculties as they were created.

The University of Berlin (Friedrich-Wilhelms Universität) was organized in 1810, when Prussia was occupied by foreign troops and reeling from the Napoleonic defeats. The Faculty of Medicine developed out of the Collegium Medico-Chirurgicum. Berlin also had an academy for training military medical officers, the Pépinière.[1] In 1818, the Faculty of Medicine was established as the Friedrich-Wilhelms Institut, interlocked with the Pépinière; students from the latter attended lectures at the Faculty of Medicine. The faculty was thereafter frequently referred to as the Pépinière.

A student enrolled at a *Gymnasium* at the age of nine or ten years. The curriculum was based on Latin and Greek, which were believed to generate flexibility in thinking as well as an appreciation of the continuing significance of antiquity. In general, the curriculum was standardized: two years in the basic sciences, followed by pathology and pharmacology, culminating in the clinical specialties. The emphasis throughout was on the lecture; direct contact with the patient did not occur until the polyclinic in the final year. Examinations began with the *Tentamen Physicium* upon completion of the basic sciences. At the end of the clinical years, the student was required to pass faculty and state examinations, in which he rarely failed. Students were considered qualified to practice medicine after their successful completion of the state examinations. The doctorate in medicine was not a requirement, but a number of Berlin graduates then spent four years in research culminating in the preparation of a dissertation (*Habilitationsschrift*) to earn a doctorate in medicine and the title *Dozent*. This title not only qualified its bearer to be a professor but also elevated his social standing.

"Freedom" was the hallmark of the life-style of the students. They attended lectures at their whim, and the sole stipulations for progress were

---

[1] *Pépinière* ("nursery") refers in general to any academy designed to train military doctors but more specifically to the institution in Berlin.

the professor's stamp in one's class book and success on the infrequent but demanding examinations. The basic-science professors complained that students who should be attending their lectures preferred to observe operations or follow the clinical lectures. At the latter, two or three students, *Praktikanten,* made a cursory examination of a patient. After asking a few superficial questions on their findings, the professor delivered a long lecture, frequently unrelated to the problems of the patient. Students were free to move from school to school, and the best students sought the most renowned teachers, who (they thought) would broaden their horizons. Vacation periods were five months long, interrupted by hospital work and military service.

Academic freedom was the hallmark of a professor's career as well. Each ruled supreme as the autocrat of his institute, and he enjoyed extended holidays in a fresh environment, devoid of academic activity, for the sake of having a "creative pause."

Mobility was also a feature of a professor's career. He frequently held his first chair in a smaller university and with success advanced to increasingly larger institutions. For most professors, election to the faculty at Berlin was the ultimate goal. The dean was a mere figurehead, who was elected by and served at the will of the faculty.

After the Franco-Prussian War, Berlin experienced a remarkable upsurge that greatly enhanced the prestige of the medical school. France paid to Prussia an indemnity of 200,000,000 francs in January 1877. This allowed the medical school to strengthen its faculty and erect new institutes. Berlin became the leading metropolis in Europe, with the world's most distinguished medical faculty.

Brief mention should be made here of some of the distinguished Berlin faculty members who would serve as mentors to Japanese students. The professor of anatomy, Karl Bogislaus Reichert (1811-1883), was, according to his students, such a zealous teacher that "he ran from one dissecting table to another" in order to direct them.[2] Wilhelm Waldeyer (1836-1921), a neuroanatomist, succeeded Reichert as director of the anatomical institute in 1883. While Reichert had been ridiculed by the students as a senile old man, Waldeyer was "an eternally youthful old man . . . an untiring pedagogical genius."[3] Oskar Hertwig (1849-1922), a reproductive biologist, was appointed to Reichert's professorship in 1888.

Emil du Bois-Reymond (1818-1896), professor of physiology and pioneer in studies of the nature of the nerve impulse, was a hero to the medical students. His lecture hall was always crowded; the students were excited, swept away by his theatrical manner and his dramatic gestures and speech. "His experiments, which he prepared in advance to the most minute detail,

---

[2] D. W. Artelt, "Die Gründung und die ersten Jahrzehnte der Berliner Medizinischen Fakultät," *Ciba Zeitschrift,* 1956, 7: 2594. Artelt excerpted descriptions of professors from the personal papers of medical students.

[3] Ibid., p. 2602.

were conducted in the manner of a priest, with conscious pompous movements celebrating high mass."[4]

The most renowned member of the faculty, Rudolf Virchow (1821-1902), founder of cellular pathology and a major figure in the rise of modern medicine, had been exiled to Würzburg in 1849 for marching with dissidents and for publishing what amounted to a manifesto for freedom and democracy. After seven years there, he was recalled to Berlin as professor of pathology and director of the Pathological Institute. Yet, among the students, Virchow "had surprisingly few enthusiastic followers even though everyone knew how important he was."[5] The students complained that he did not prepare his lectures carefully and that he had little regard for his students, who deserved more than his fame."[6]

The area of internal medicine was dominated by Professor K. F. Theodor von Frerichs (1814-1885), physician in chief at La Charité and a founder of experimental pathology. He succeeded Schönlein, the last great bedside teacher, in 1859 and was himself a superb teacher, his "lectures logically organized, describing with great eloquence varieties of symptoms. He developed the diagnosis with great clarity."[7]

As in most faculties, relationships were not always harmonious. Frerichs's career was blighted by the aggressive enmity of Virchow, and Frerichs was openly hostile to Ludwig Traube, who held the second chair in medicine. One faction of the faculty was led by Virchow, Du Bois-Reymond, and Traube, while Frerichs and Reichert were the strongest voices in the opposition.

Ludwig Traube (1818-1876) was appointed to the faculty in 1857, as a specialist in pulmonary diseases and an investigator of the relationship of the vagus nerve to pulmonary function. Friedrich Trendelenburg (1844-1924), professor of surgery in Berlin and pioneer in operations for pulmonary embolism, commented on Traube, "At the age of forty-seven years, he looked older than his age, serious, intelligent, [with] somewhat piercing eyes and a fat ball of cotton in each ear."[8]

Moritz Heinrich Romberg (1795-1873), who wrote the first formal textbook on nervous diseases, *Lehrbuch der Nervenkrankheiten* (1840-46), taught neuropsychiatry from 1838 to 1865. His successor, Wilhelm Griesinger, (1817-1868), launched his scientific study of mental illness, a field that continued to be dominated by German scientists for many years. Carl Friedrich Otto Westphal (1833-1890) succeeded Griesinger in 1868.

The professor of surgery, Bernhard von Langenbeck (1810-1887), appointed in 1847, made his principal contributions in orthopedic and plastic surgery. Like other surgeons, he had a compulsion for beginning his day at

[4] Ibid., p. 2595.
[5] Ibid.
[6] Ibid.
[7] Ibid., pp. 2595-96.
[8] Ibid., p. 2596.

dawn, and his course in operative surgery started shortly after six o'clock. No student missed his lectures, which he held in "a small morgue teeming with flies and crowded with students."[9] Langenbeck's motto was *Nunquam retrorsum* ("Never backwards"). The only recollection of the students concerning his predecessor, Schlemm, was that his lectures were interrupted by his great puffs on a fat cigar and sips from a stein of beer.

Johann Christian Jüngken (1793-1875), professor of surgery until 1868, was another member of the Virchow faction. He had become a *Privatdozent* at the age of twenty-four and remained a member of the faculty for four decades. He disputed with the professor of obstetrics, Eduard Martin (1809-1875), over the boundaries between surgery and gynecology—who should perform mastectomies and who should perform pelvic surgery. The hostility was so strong that Jüngken refused to allow Martin to use his operating room.

There was no mandatory retirement age, but as Jüngken approached his seventy-fifth birthday, his colleagues assumed that he would retire. At a festive dinner in his honor, they gave many laudatory speeches, but after all the words of adulation, Jüngken announced that he had no intention of retiring. However, he did retire in October 1868 and was succeeded by Adolf Bardeleben (1819-1895). A student of the great Johannes Mueller, Bardeleben was one of the first surgeons to carry out fundamental research. The students described him as "patriarchal in appearance but earthy in manner."[10]

Jüngken also fought over the relationship between ophthalmology and surgery, and it was not until he retired that the two were separated, when Albrecht von Graefe (1828-1870) was named professor. He ushered in the modern era of ophthalmic surgery.

Karl Gustav Mitscherlich (1805-1871), a pioneer in experimental pharmacology, held that professorship from 1849 until his death. On the basis of his personal observations and his valuable private collection of drugs, he wrote a textbook of pharmacology, which went through a number of editions. Mitscherlich was succeeded by Oskar Liebreich (1839-1908), who prepared the first modern soporific, chloral hydrate.

Ernst von Leyden (1832-1910), successor to Frerichs, was a student of nervous disorders and to his students "the elegant, polished man of the world, certainly a great physician, but at the time had already passed his peak."[11] The German school of pediatrics was founded in Berlin by Eduard Heinrich Henoch (1820-1910) and Carl A.J.C. Gerhardt (1833-1902). Henoch is best-known for his description of allergic nonthrombocytopenic purpura. Gerhardt succeeded Traube in 1885, and Henoch was forced to retire in 1893 because of a detached retina. Gerhardt's *Handbuch der Kinderkrankheiten* in sixteen volumes (1877-93) was a pediatrician's favorite

[9]Ibid., p. 2597.
[10]Ibid., p. 2599.
[11]Ibid., p. 2602.

reference source. The students described him as having "a fiery red face and apoplectic constitution—a propadeutic pedant—a fine diagnostician and a therapeutic nihilist."[12]

When a proposal was put forward by J. Otto Heubner, who was elected to the chair in pediatrics in December 1893, to make pediatrics a separate department, the proposed division was bitterly attacked by Virchow at Heubner's first faculty meeting. Nevertheless, the proposal was endorsed, and thus the first department of pediatrics was established in Berlin.

Probably the greatest disappointment for the faculty came with the election of a new professor of surgery in 1882. They had unanimously voted to invite the renowned gastrointestinal surgeon Theodor Billroth (1829-1894) of Vienna to succeed Bernhard Langenbeck as professor of surgery. But Billroth was content in Vienna as a member of the Austrian House of Lords, an intimate friend of Johannes Brahms, and a leader of the intellectual and artistic circles of the city.

Robert Koch (1843-1910) joined the staff of the Imperial Health Department in Berlin on July 10, 1881, and one year later announced the discovery of the tubercle bacillus. Koch found teaching a burdensome interference with his research, and the students saw little of him. He left the faculty in 1891 to become director of the Institute of Infectious Diseases. Henceforth, he concentrated his efforts at his new institute, where he continued to make his great discoveries.

Germany was the last major European nation to establish a firm base in Japan. The first German move in this direction was made by August Luehdorf, who came to Hakodate and Shimoda on the German ship *Greta*, July 4, 1855.[13] Luehdorf submitted an appeal to the shogunate that Prussia be granted the same rights of commerce as were enjoyed by America, Britain, Holland, and France. But the response was negative because the *Greta*, which was under charter, was flying the American flag and Luehdorf was considered an imposter.

It was not until 1860 that Count Fritz Eulenburg led the first official Prussian mission to establish trade and relations in the Orient. The Berlin government was eager to expand its foreign markets in East Asia, particularly in Bangkok, Edo, and Peking. Prussia feared that "the treaties which England, France, and America had concluded with China, Japan, and Siam would possibly move those empires to grant less favorable treatment to nationals and ships of other countries."[14]

The Eulenburg mission was prepared with characteristic German thoroughness and included Ferdinand von Richthofen, geologist; Gustav Spiess, economist; and Maximilian August Scipio von Brandt, diplomatic

---

[12] Ibid.

[13] Kurt Meissner, *Deutsche in Japan, 1639-1939* (Stuttgart and Berlin: Deutsche Verlags-Anstalt, 1940), p. 22.

[14] M. S. von Brandt, *Dreiunddreissig Jahre in Ost-Asiens. Erinnerungen eines deutschen Diplomats* (Leipzig: Georg Wigand, 1906), vol. 1, p. 8.

attaché. The four ships of the expedition sailed in the winter of 1859, via England, the Cape of Good Hope, and Singapore, with Brandt on the Prussian warship *Arkona.* They rode out a typhoon off the Japanese coast and landed at Edo on September 8, 1859.

A temporary residence was found in Tokyo at Akabane, Shiba Park, the former *yashiki* of the *daimyo* of Kii *han,* on a lovely peninsula near Osaka. The Prussians were unaccustomed to the cold and drafty Japanese houses, and their discomfort was increased by the voracius goat they had brought along for a milk supply: he devoured the paper windows in their house, and they gave him to the first Japanese who would accept him. Within a few days the Prussians moved into an official residence in Yokohama, hoisted the Prussian flag, and shocked their Japanese attendants by not removing their shoes while in the house.

They relied on interpreters, all of whom were Dutch. The complex procedure of communicating began with the Dutch interpreter translating from German to Dutch, after which a Japanese translated from Dutch to Japanese. The principal interpreter for the Prussians was Henry Heusken, a young Hollander who had been lent to them by the American consul, Townsend Harris.

In negotiating a commercial treaty, Eulenburg not only faced a deteriorating shogunate but was speaking as well for a disunited Germany. In the minds of the Japanese, "Prussia" equalled "Germany," and when Eulenburg tried to add other German states to the treaty, it was declined. The Japanese-Prussian treaty was signed January 24, 1861, but not ratified until January 21, 1864.

Once the treaty was signed, Eulenburg left Japan, and Consul Max von Brandt became the leader of the mission in Japan. The son of August Heinrich von Brandt, a Prussian general and analyst of military affairs, Max von Brandt at first followed his father's military career. He completed preparatory studies at the outstanding *Französisches Gymnasium* in Berlin and graduated from the military academy. But at the conclusion of his studies, he entered a career in foreign diplomacy and in 1859 was sent to Japan as attaché on the East Asia expedition. After successive promotions he was designated consul general in 1866 and ambassador to Japan in 1872.

The permanent Prussian consulate, which he established in the legation settlement in Yokohama, lay about halfway between Kanagawa and the foreign colony. It was simple in design and surrounded by the traditional charming Japanese garden.

The pioneer German commercial firms at Yokohama were smaller than their British and American counterparts. Their major exports were raw silk and silkworms, with smaller amounts of copper, tea, plants, and other native products. Imports, on the other hand, were quite small and limited largely to textiles and metals.

The Yokohama foreign community in the 1860s was dominated by British and Americans. With access bridges closely guarded and protection assured by surrounding canals, life in the community became pleasant. An unknown author described it in 1863: "A beautiful quay has been built where, in the evening, one sees elegant ladies strolling about. . . . The place is turning into a miniature Paris. The gentlemen wear patent-leather shoes and elegant gloves and would wrinkle their noses if they were to encounter one of the settlers in a flannel shirt without a high-button collar or gloves."[15]

Until 1863, the Prussians with their small staff remained officially under the protection and jurisdiction of the British. Furthermore, since essentially all of the banks, insurance agencies, and shipping officials were British, the Prussians found it necessary to adopt English as their language of exchange. The Japanese were delighted to find that three of the Western powers, Britain, America, and Germany, used a common language.

An important rallying point for the Germans was the Germania Club, founded in Yokohama in 1863 on property made available by the Japanese government. Gildermeister of the Kniffen Trading Company and Consul von Brandt, who were the founders, gave as its raison d'être "to prove expressly that every one of us is proud to be a member of the German nation."[16] The small German community was closely knit: as the historian Meissner has put it, "Thus the Germans in Japan achieved unification under Prussian leadership, eight years before Versailles and even before the War of 1866."[17]

The social life of the Germans in Yokohama was limited. They complained over (among other things) the high cost of alcoholic beverages and the complete absence of ice. In another area, if a foreigner wished to take a Japanese woman to his quarters for lovemaking, an authorization from the Japanese Customs Office was mandatory, and when intercourse was completed, the woman had to return to the Customs Office and report her earnings.

During the final fifteen years (1854-68) of Tokugawa rule, at least 200 foreign technologists and language teachers worked in Japan. The majority were members of official military, naval, and technical missions. Of the 200, more than 80 were French; about 60, Dutch; 30, from the United Kingdom; and the remainder, Germans and Americans. The foreign employees were known as *O-yatoi gaikokujin* ("honorable foreign menial") or simply *yatoi.*

The advantage of employing *yatoi* was first pointed out to the Japanese by the French minister Léon Roches in 1864, but it was the aggressive Sir Harry Parkes who in 1867 recognized the full opportunity for exercising

[15] Meissner, *Deutsche in Japan,* p. 31.
[16] Ibid., p. 40.
[17] Ibid., p. 39.

influence that this practice gave to foreign powers. Thus, Great Britain left the French and other countries far behind in this regard. Parkes repeatedly seized initiatives; when, for example, in 1873 an informal understanding had been reached for the Americans to build railways, Parkes convinced the Japanese that British skills were superior. American influence was limited not only by her involvement in the Civil War, but also by a consular act of 1856 that barred American diplomats from recommending U. S. nationals for foreign service. (Most of the Americans in Japan were there ostensibly to teach English and to learn Japanese.)

In the first year of the Meiji era, the concept of employing foreigners under contract with the Meiji government was firmly established. Medicine, language skills, and natural sciences were the major fields in which they were used. The government's goal throughout the *yatoi* era was to educate Japanese as rapidly as possible to replace the foreign employees.

There had been only a few German employees during the *Bakumatsu* (end of the *Bakufu* years). Therefore, on December 10, 1867, Ambassador Brandt pressed the Japanese government to implement Article 21 of the treaty with Prussia. It called for German to be a major foreign language, for Japanese students to study in Prussia, and for the opening of a language school to teach German to Japanese youths. Brandt stressed that Japanese students should be studying in Prussia as well as in Holland, France, and Britain. His protestations were heeded, and the following year he was granted funds for bringing the first teachers from Prussia.

Containment of foreigners within the areas of the open ports had been an avowed policy but one not stricly enforced since the *Bakufu* period. The foreign powers had full jurisdiction over their nationals, including those employed by the Meiji government. The Japanese found this arrangement distasteful. All foreigners were required to reside in *kyoryuchi,* special restricted areas. (This regulation was not strictly enforced, and in fact the majority of foreigners preferred to live outside the *kyoryuchi.*) Japanese could not rent or purchase houses or other buildings in these areas. They were prepared and provided by the government, and all structures were owned by the government or by private Japanese entrepreneurs. *O-yatoi* were required to carry at all times a work and travel permit, which bore the seal of *Gaimusho* (the foreign ministry).

Foreigners employed by the Japanese government were paid in dollars Mex rather than in the fluctuating local currency.[18] Although the Japanese opened a mint in May 1871 and officially adopted the gold standard, Mexican silver continued to be used at the treaty ports.

[18]Mexican and Peruvian silver pesos were introduced to the Orient on the Manila galleons sailing between Acapulco and Manila annually beginning in 1565. As the richest ships that sailed the oceans, they carried the silver pesos primarily to trade for silk and other Oriental luxuries with Chinese merchants from Macao. The silver pesos became known as "dollars Mex" and were the currency of the seaports of China and Japan.

The employment of *O-yatoi* peaked in 1874 and 1875 with over 800 for each of those years. By 1877, the number diminished to 500-600 and then leveled off at about 200 employees a year.[19]

Upon the Japanese government's decision in 1870 to adopt German medicine, eleven Japanese students were sent to Germany for postgraduate medical studies. The most important of them was Osawa Kenji (1852-1927), who studied muscle-nerve physiology in the laboratories of Hermann von Helmholtz and Emil Du Bois-Reymond. Another, Nagai Nagayoshi, studied pharmacology at Berlin and remained there for an indefinite period. The other students included Yamawaki Gen, anatomy; Iwasa Shin (or Imai Gen), physiology and physics; Sagara Gentei, pathology; and Ikeda Kensai, surgery, especially military medicine.

When Ambassador Brandt received the Japanese request on March 18, 1870, for two German teachers of medicine, he recommended to the Berlin government that they should be military men, "because military medical officers would, by nature of their status, be regarded in all circles with the highest esteem, would be accepted by the aristocracy, and might even become personal physicians to his majesty the *Tenno.*"[20] Benjamin Karl Leopold Mueller (1824-1893), *Oberstabsarzt*, was the man selected to lead the German medical mission.

Born on July 24, 1824, in Mainz, Hesse, Mueller studied medicine in Bonn from 1842 to 1844 and then in Berlin, where he graduated in February 1847. He then trained in surgery at La Charité, where his thesis for the doctorate in medicine reported on his studies in surgery. After earning a commission in the army medical corps, Mueller taught at the Pépinière.

Mueller explained his selection for the mission to Japan by his years of service on a similar mission in Haiti. In 1858 he had arrived in Port-au-Prince to serve as a government medical officer. Torn by repeated revolutions and assassinations since her successful revolt against French rule (1794), the island was in a primitive condition, afflicted with disease and starvation. Smallpox had reached Haiti, then called Hispaniola, in 1518, and epidemics broke out repeatedly. The first slave ship from Africa brought malaria and yellow fever at the beginning of French rule in 1697. No public-health measures were instituted until 1847, under a medical/sanitary board, the *Jury Médical*, but its actions were inadequate and ineffectual. A program to train medical practitioners was begun in 1808, and in 1844 Haiti's President Philippe Guerrier proposed that it be reorganized on the American pattern. But a revolution in early 1844, by which Santo

---

[19]For further information on *O-yatoi*, see Hazel J. Jones, *Monumenta Nopponica*, 1978, *33* (1-2): 9-30; R. S. Schwantes, "Foreign Employees in the Development of Japan" (unpublished manuscript), and Hazel J. Jones, *The Meiji Government and Foreign Employees, 1868-1900*, Doctoral Dissertation, University of Michigan, 1967.

[20]Benjamin Carl Leopold Mueller, "Tokio Igaku: Skizzen und Erinnerungen aus der Zeit des geistigen Umschwungs in Japan, 1871-1876," *Deutsche Rundschau*, 1888, *57*: 316.

Domingo gained independence, thwarted any such attempts. President
N. Fabré Geffrard, who held office from 1859 until his exile in 1867, made
another effort to reorganize and strengthen the school, and Mueller became
the leader of this reform. On his return to Berlin in 1867, Mueller was sent
to East Prussia to control an epidemic of typhus and to conduct a general
evaluation of health problems.

As his deputy on the Japan mission Mueller chose Theodor Hoffmann,
who had studied medicine in Breslau and also graduated in Berlin. He
trained in internal medicine at La Charité with Ludwig Traube (1818-1876)
and then served in the imperial navy.

The conditions of their employment were articulated at a preliminary
conference in Tokyo attended by Brandt; Sawa Nobuyoshi, the minister of
foreign affairs; and Matsudaira Yoshinaga, the Japanese director of the
existing medical school. Mueller and Hoffmann were to be attached to the
German legation but would deal directly with the Japanese *Mombusho*
(ministry of education). They would have complete authority in all educational matters, including the selection of medical students, and would be
the direct superiors of all Japanese and foreigners employed by the school.
(Financial matters and the conduct of the students were to be the responsibility of the Japanese director.) Mueller considered this independence
essential to the success of the mission.

The outbreak of the Franco-Prussian War on July 19, 1870, delayed
their departure, and Mueller feared their mission would be abandoned.
Shortly after the treaty of peace was signed in Frankfurt on May 10, 1871,
however, they were directed to prepare to sail, and one month later they
left for Japan by way of New York. After a leisurely month-long trans-
continental tour with stops at Niagara Falls, Omaha, and Salt Lake City,
they embarked at San Francisco. Their vessel, the *America,* arrived at
Yokohama on August 23.

Iwasa Jun, the first Japanese representative to welcome Mueller and
Hoffman, visited them in Yokohama within a few days. He expressed
gratitude for the successful outcome of the recommendation he and Sagara
Chian had submitted two years earlier. Mueller and Hoffmann then made a
round of courtesy calls, culminating in an audience with the *Tenno,*
Emperor Meiji.

They staged their first visit to the school as a Prussian military parade.
In full dress uniform crowned with spiked helmets, and preceded by a
caparisoned German cavalry detachment, Mueller and Hoffmann rode
through the gate of the Todo *yashiki.* They found in the center a group of
spacious buildings with wide porches, tile roofs, and sliding paper doors or
screens (*shoji*) as external walls. On the periphery were smaller, shedlike
structures along drainage ditches filled with foul water. There was a
dilapidated garden, surrounded by a high wall.

Mueller made a brief address on the nature of their mission; it was
translated by Shiba Ryokai, who taught medicine at the school. They were

officially greeted by Sato Shochu, who had just succeeded Iwasa Jun as the Japanese director. The student supervisors, Ishiguro Tadanori and Hasegawa Yasushi, stood at his side.

The improvised classrooms were a striking contrast to the splendid halls in which they had studied at Bonn and Berlin:

About 300 students were introduced to us. They were sitting in a series of halls with ten to sixteen at a table. Each student had his *hibachi* [small heater] and his pipe beside him. They were reading aloud from books, which appertained for the most part to some scientific field. But they read different chapters and the books were in different languages. All of them were reading at the same time in the well-known Oriental sing-song manner, so that one had the impression he was entering a synagogue. Japanese overseers, who also had *hibachis,* pipes, and cups of tea, sat at the larger tables. Their chief task was to assure that the students read loudly and without any pause and to explain, if possible, passages to the students. But they understood most of them no better than did their students.[21]

As soon as a student had acquired superficial knowledge of a foreign language, he would pretend to read any book recommended by his teacher; the thickest were the most popular. The Japanese staff based their evaluation of the students solely on the number of pages read: "This one went through two hundred pages of anatomy; that student read the entire pathology text and the other read it twice." Many students were attempting to read specialized texts that were beyond the abilities of a German medical student.[22]

Before coming to Igakujo, the students had usually spent several years as apprentices to medical practitioners, and the school was regarded as nothing more than a supplement to that apprenticeship—as Mueller described it, ". . . a place to satisfy one's curiosity in regard to certain anatomical facts." There were no teaching schedules and students were not required to attend classes—they came and went as they wished. The interaction between students and their teachers consisted largely of irrelevant questions asked and meaningless answers given. Mueller's low opinion of the medical students derived from the fact that "a great number of men unfit for any other profession took up medical studies, and furthermore many of the students of this school were already far advanced in age and incapable of any intellectual pursuits as a result of their many years of Chinese education."[23]

Devoted to the tradition of freedom and solitude to which a German professor was accustomed, Mueller projected a schedule that included four hours of lecture a day with the remaining time to be used as he saw fit. The Japanese were dismayed; they had expected him to be at the school from eight o'clock in the morning until five in the evening in order to be

[21] Ibid., pp. 318-19.
[22] Ibid., p. 319.
[23] Ibid., pp. 321-22.

always available to the staff and students. They had assumed that Mueller and Hoffmann would be able to lecture on any subject at any time and without any preparation. Instead, Mueller's daily schedule included four hours of lecture and clinical instruction, three to four hours in preparation for teaching and administrative tasks, and one and a half hours to instruct the interpreters, with a similar amount of time for the study of Japanese. In addition, he was frequently called upon to care for patients. It soon became necessary for Mueller to limit his house calls to ones he made to high officials of the emperor's court and their families. All other patients seeking his personal care were asked to come to his polyclinic at the hospital so that he could use them for teaching.

The *yashiki* was markedly unsuited for use as a teaching facility or a hospital: "The inner buildings consisted of a series of large and relatively low halls, and many small rooms for concubines, singers, dancing girls, and attendants." Slops and other refuse were tossed indiscriminately into ponds and ditches, and, as Mueller commented wryly, "with the stagnant waters they form as many breeding grounds for infectious diseases as there are inner courts." Any efforts to introduce sanitary practices and hygiene in the hospital were frustrated by the continuing custom that patients' families moved in with them, bringing servants, clothing, and bedding, as well as cooking equipment, charcoal, and food. The patient, the family, their servants, and all their paraphernalia were stuffed into a single, poorly ventilated room, where everyone ate and slept. But custom could not be revoked, and Mueller commented: "We would have no patients had we not accepted their families." With only the flimsy *shoji* as external walls and only *hibachi* as sources of heat, by midwinter the temperature of the classroom (-8 to $-10°$ Celsius) dropped near to that outside. Mueller's fingers became so stiff from the cold that in order to perform surgery he dipped them repeatedly into a kettle of hot water both before and during an operation.[24]

The Japanese agreed with Mueller that the *yashiki* could not serve as a hospital, and they gave high priority to the construction of a new facility. They asked him to design a replica of a leading European hospital as "a temple of Aesculapius whose dome would illuminate with electric beams all of Tokyo—a huge European monument with the newest ventilation, heating, and facilities."[25]

Since such a structure would have required the services of European architects and many years to complete, Mueller designed a more practical facility, with the medical school as the main building and two adjoining rooms of barracks to serve as a hospital and to house the pharmacy, housekeeping, and other services. The exterior would harmonize with Japanese architectural design, except that doors and windows would replace the porous *shoji* and the interior would follow a European pattern.

[24] Ibid.
[25] Ibid., p. 328.

The entire project was suddenly dropped, however, and Mueller discovered that the Japanese were not sincere in their plans for a lavish hospital project; these were only a contrivance to help them realize their intention of adopting Western medicine as rapidly as possible. Efforts were then directed toward improving the *yashiki*. The *shoji* were replaced by panes of glass for better illumination and protection, benches and desks replaced *tatami*, and stoves were installed so that students no longer shivered by their *hibachi*. Two lecture halls were erected, one for the basic sciences and the other for clinical lectures.

Interpreters were essential, but only one competent person was available. He was Miyake Hiizu (1848-1938), son of Miyake Gonsai, a leading *Rangakusha*, and had lived with an American missionary, J. C. Hepburn, for four years. As a result of this background, he had gained reasonable proficiency in English as well as some understanding of medicine and its terminology.[26]

A small army of Japanese were introduced to Mueller as officials, teachers, aides, and servants—all of them were said to be there to work for the new teachers from Germany. But only a few of them were of any use; the best was Taguchi Kazuyoshi, who had some knowledge of medicine and who became an excellent prosector in the anatomy laboratory.[27] Mueller deduced that save for Taguchi and a few others, the purpose of the staff was to spy, not only on the German teachers but on each other. He would have nothing to do with them and insisted that he and Hoffmann select and train their own assistants.

A further cause of frustration to him was the antagonism of the older Japanese physicians and officials, who opposed him at every opportunity because they were jealous of his superior knowledge as well as that of his students.

Mueller heaped Teutonic scorn on Kaiseijo; he found especially galling the Japanese suggestion that he should use it as his model for the medical school. In Mueller's view, Verbeck, the director, was "an American missionary trained as a plumber and obsequious to any whim of the Japanese authorities."[28] The teaching staff was a disorganized mélange of "people from all professions and nations possible . . . a traveling salesman and a beer brewer, pharmacists, sailors, naval architects. At one time serious consideration was given to hiring a circus clown as a teacher of physical education. . . . A clown from the same circus had been hired as a teacher of foreign languages. . . . Any unemployed foreigner with no ability whatsoever could be almost certain of obtaining a teaching post at Kaiseijo."[29]

In his opinion, the teaching program was as disorderly and unregulated as was the staff. A Swiss and then a Dane had taught German; the former

---

[26] Miyake later studied medicine in Germany and became professor of pathology and medical history at the school in 1882.

[27] Taguchi also studied later in Berlin and became professor of anatomy.

[28] Mueller, "Tokio Igaku," p. 446.

[29] Ibid., p. 445.

could neither read nor write correctly, and both spoke with heavy native accents. Because of its slipshod program, the foreign community described Kaiseijo derisively as the "asylum for lost souls."[30]

Mueller's criticism of Kaiseijo was to some extent justified. During the turbulent years associated with the fall of the Tokugawa, the school had been neglected. It was taken over by the new Meiji government in 1869 and renamed Nanko (south school), but it continued to be referred to as Kaiseijo. Its educational emphasis was on languages—English, Dutch, and French—and it attracted some good students. Some of the school's graduates went on to distinguished and influential careers as intellectual leaders. Unfortunately, Mueller was unaware of the efforts to revitalize Kaiseijo. The school was just entering a period of transition when he formed his evaluation.

The teaching materials Mueller found at the *yashiki* were minimal —parts of a dilapidated skeleton and a few Auzoux papier-mâché anatomical models.[31] The few outdated medical texts were in Dutch or English, with just a single German text, Bock's *Buch von gesunden und kranken Menschen*. The Germans improvised other teaching materials, only to unearth after a number of months a more than adequate supply of texts, skeletons, and instruments. These had been stored in crates near an access area so that they could be removed immediately in case of an outbreak of one of the frequent fires that ravaged Tokyo. Among them were five complete and well-preserved skeletons with skulls, anatomical models and charts, microscopes, texts, and ophthalmological instruments. All had been crated for so long, without any record of the contents, that not one member of the Japanese staff knew of their existence.

Despite Joseph Siddall's efforts in 1868 to establish a proper pharmacy, Mueller found an utter jumble. Ingredients for prescriptions were in jars that were labelled incorrectly or had no labels whatsoever. Since medications were purchased from unscrupulous dealers in order to get the lowest price, one could not be sure that the material purchased was that which had been requested. The men who worked in the pharmacy were untrained and could read only Japanese labels. The sole reliable foreign pharmacy was in Yokohama. Niewirth, a professional pharmacist from Germany, was brought to Tokyo and converted the disorganized dispensary to the first modern hospital pharmacy in Japan.

Sato Shochu and his Japanese colleagues wished to assign the older students to advanced standing, but Mueller refused to do so until he had evaluated each student's knowledge of anatomy, physiology, pathology, and surgery. Eight days after his arrival in Yokohama, therefore, Mueller examined the nineteen students the Japanese had nominated as being the

---

[30] Ibid., p. 21.

[31] Named for L.T.J. Auzoux (1797-1880) of Paris, whose models were widely used to teach anatomy, especially when cadavers were not available. They were referred to as "artificial anatomies."

best of a total of about three hundred. The results were as he had anticipated: "Not one of them was prepared in anatomy and physiology; not one of them could describe the circulation of the blood (although more than one of them had studied cardiology); not one was able to identify the right and the left thigh and explain the reason for his choice."[32]

The students' limited anatomical nomenclature was in Chinese, and the terms were based on speculation rather than on actual dissection. As an example, the word for ligament, *kinmyaku*, was applied to any structure —blood vessel, nerve, or lymph duct—that vaguely resembled a ligament.

Mueller would have preferred to postpone instruction until the students had completed their premedical training, but he accepted the fact that for practical purposes he was obliged to begin classes without any delay, in order to maintain the confidence and support of the Japanese. As soon as the students learned that a new educational program was to be introduced, about half of them departed.

Mueller gave his opening lecture, in osteology, on September 4, 1871. After completing that course, he taught anatomy, and Hoffmann, physiology. In an effort to accelerate the educational program and make it more attractive, they added lectures in bandaging, pharmacology, and the examination of patients. But when it became clear to them that the students were unable to learn the additional subjects, they discontinued them.

The language of instruction was determined by the language that the interpreter spoke—German or English. Mueller and Hoffmann used carefully prepared manuscripts and printed all medical terms in large block letters on the blackboard. The interpreter translated the lecture sentence by sentence, and after class the manuscript was distributed to the students. Mueller also compiled his lectures with annotated references for purchase by the students.

In the afternoon, the best students explained the lecture to the others. Each Saturday the students were examined on the material presented in the lectures during the previous week. Hoffmann followed the same procedure in physiology. Because they had always learned by rote, the students found learning the large number of terms easy; but independent, conceptual thinking was completely alien to them. Although the Oriental tradition was to accept a teacher's statements without question, the students were deeply suspicious of their foreign mentors and seized any opportunity to prove them wrong by asking tricky questions.

At the end of December, the minister of education, Oki Takato (1831-1899), agreed that the number of students permitted to continue should be determined by an examination. The majority of the students failed; fifty-nine continued. Subsequent withdrawals for health and other reasons left the class with a total of thirty-five students.

The need for student assistants fluent in German became more pressing, and Mueller selected the six most promising candidates, to whom

[32]Mueller, "Tokio Igaku," p. 142.

he gave personal instruction for one and a half hours each day. This was a challenging project because the only available text was a grammar for teaching German to English-speaking people. It was necessary, therefore, to find an English-speaking interpreter to translate the grammar into Japanese; the students then translated the Japanese text into German.

After a few months Mueller and Hoffmann became convinced that because of the students' ignorance of chemistry, biology, and physics, as well as of German, a preparatory program was imperative. He asked Ambassador Brandt to arrange with the Berlin government for sending qualified teachers in these subjects. At the same time Mueller decided that no new students would be accepted until the preparatory school was in operation.

The Japanese recommended two men, whom Mueller described as a beer brewer and a salesman, to teach the premedical subjects. It was only after heated arguments that he was able to employ two Germans, a Dr. Simmons and a Mr. Wagner, on a temporary basis until the new faculty arrived. Simmons had studied at Kiel and Tübingen and had come to Japan just before the outbreak of the Franco-Prussian War. His original commission was as advisor on the construction of a European-style hospital, until Mueller came, Wagner had been wasting his talents teaching chemistry, mathematics, and physics in an inferior secondary school.

Mueller's heavy teaching load was lightened when in 1872 Friedrich Karl Wilhelm Donitz (1838-1912) came to teach anatomy at Igakujo. He remained there for three years, from 1872 to 1875. Then, after a financial dispute, he left Tokyo for the interior of Japan, where he devoted himself to practical problems of sanitation and disease control. When civil war broke out in 1877, Donitz cared for casualties at the hospital. A lifelong student of entomology and a skilled artist, he not only amassed a fine collection of specimens but also illustrated his own publications. Following a brief trip to Europe in 1880, he returned to southern Japan to live at Saga until his recall to Berlin in 1886. There he worked with Koch and with Ehrlich, pursuing both his entomological and his public-health research, and wrote many works on parasitology.

In January 1872 the medical school was awarded a legal charter and its name changed from Igakujo (also Toko) to Daiichi Daigaku-ku Igakko (number-one university medical school). Sato Shochu retired in August 1872 to become director of Juntendo Hospital, and Hasegawa Yasushi (also Tai), served in the interim until Sagara Chian, who was also director of the new medical bureau in *Mombusho,* assumed the post on October 8, 1872. Hasegawa had been recommended as dean at Nagasaki but chose to remain at Igakujo.

The first premedical teachers arrived in March 1873: Franz Martin Hilgendorf (8139-1904), who had been *Dozent* of zoology at the Leopold Academy in Dresden, to teach botany and zoology; Hermann Cochius,

Table 1. The Curriculum

First Year—Third Preparatory Class: German, arithmetic, general geography, Japanese and Chinese studies. (Students who had completed a comparable course in a German school were not required to enroll in this class.)

Second Year—Second Preparatory Class: German, geometry, geography, history, medical Latin, introduction to natural sciences.

Third Year—First Preparatory Class: Scientific German, Latin, mathematics, chemistry, physics, and natural sciences.

Fourth Year: Anatomy, German, German composition, Latin, mathematics, chemistry, physics, and natural sciences.

Fifth Year: Dissection, physiology, general surgery, laboratory experiments, histology, natural sciences, chemistry, and physics.

Sixth Year: General and social pathology, therapeutics, pharmacology, surgical specialties, operative surgery, and methods of clinical examination.

Seventh Year: Surgical and medical polyclinic, physical examination, surgical anatomy, surgical specialties, and ophthalmology.

Eighth Year: Polyclinics in all subjects, hospital assignments, and lecture-reviews of major subjects.

from a secondary school in Berlin, to teach mathematics, physics, and chemistry; and Hermann Funk, a language teacher from Berlin, to teach Latin and Greek. They were joined in July by one Holtz, to teach geography and history. The preparatory staff was completed a few months later with the arrival of one Lange, another philologist from Berlin, to teach foreign languages, and one Schendel, also from Berlin, for mathematics.

Mueller recommended to the Japanese that the preparatory school be converted to a complete German *Gymnasium* offering a broader, superior education. The course would be of seven years' duration, with instruction in the sciences, modern languages, and Latin. After completing his studies at the *Gymnasium,* a student would spend five years in the medical school, followed by three years in a postgraduate medical faculty in Germany. The Japanese government refused to adopt this proposal, however, on the grounds that implementing the program would take too many years to complete. Some years later Mueller learned to his amusement and satisfaction that his entire proposal was adopted and implemented in 1886.

After the preparatory school had been adequately staffed, Mueller established a seven-year curriculum, with an eighth year for practical training on the hospital wards and in the polyclinic. The first three years were designated for premedical courses, followed by four years of clinical instruction. A comprehensive examination was given at the end of the hospital and polyclinical year.

The educational philosophy and the curriculum imitated the Germanic model. The German language was taught throughout the three preparatory years and in the first year of the medical curriculum; there was no instruction in any other modern foreign language.

This emphasis on German required that after three years a student must be able to follow lectures without an interpreter and after five years to express himself clearly and precisely in German, both orally and in writing. Mueller defended the exclusive use of German on the grounds that learning more than one foreign language would have been too difficult. He acknowledged that English or French could have been chosen as the language of the school but pointed out the significance of a mastery of German for postgraduate programs: "The number of good European institutions for continuing medical studies in the German language is far greater than [that] in any other language, and no country has a richer wealth of excellent translations of valuable works than Germany."[33]

That the Japanese had become increasingly aware of this fact since Mueller's departure was confirmed by a statement included in the 1883-1884 calendar of the school: "Since today the natural sciences and the literary arts of Europe may be studied with the greatest breadth and depth in Germany, it is essential that students master German in order to be able to pursue such studies from German texts."

The students underwent a ritualistic annual public examination before members of the German diplomatic delegation and high officials of the Japanese government. One such occasion was adorned by the presence of the *Tenno,* which gave great pride and pleasure to Mueller as well as to his German and Japanese colleagues. At the successful completion of his studies, the student received a diploma that declared him qualified to fill any medical post in Japan.

Once the design of the curriculum was established, criteria were developed for the selection of the students. Age, preliminary education, and physical condition were the major considerations.

1. An age requirement of fourteen to sixteen years: Since birth records were unknown in Japan, age was estimated on the basis of physical and intellectual development. Moreover, an applicant's statement on his age had to be adjusted, since an infant was considered to be one year old at birth. Furthermore, the Japanese New Year, which was calculated on a lunar basis, occurred eight to ten weeks after the European year began.

2. A basic Chinese-Japanese education commensurate with the age of the applicant: This was continued in the first preparatory-school year because a knowledge of Chinese was considered the mark of an educated man.

3. A strong physical condition with no impairment of the sense organs: Mueller deemed this stipulation important because the practice of medicine had historically been a haven for the physically and mentally unfit.

Most of the students paid a tuition fee; those who could not afford to do so were required to enter government medical service after graduation and repay the debt. The minimum time spent in the service was usually five years.

[33] Ibid., p. 449.

After just two years, Theodor Hoffmann predicted a rosy future for the school. After tracing its development since 1871, he noted that thus far European medicine had exerted a minimal influence on Japanese medicine: "but it is reasonable to expect good results and broader influence in the course of one decade, considering the excellent capacity of the Japanese for learning, and that arrangements have now been made to give them the necessary foundations in science and language."[34]

Some Japanese traditions and customs were both perplexing and frustrating to the foreigners. Adoption of boys in order to insure that the family name be continued was a common practice at all social levels. A merchant might adopt his chief clerk in order to give him a personal interest in the firm. Thus one might find a family drawn from five or six sources, with no kinship ties, calling each other father and son, mother and daughter, brother and sister.

Several medical students tried to use the practice of adoption to avoid payment of the tuition fee. As an example, Mueller cited the case of the second-year student who asked to be placed in the tuition-free category. Investigations revealed that his parents were under no financial stress, and the request was denied. Undaunted, the student arranged to be adopted by a married couple of low economic status who were unable to pay the tuition fee. Mueller then had no choice but to cancel the required payment.

Although attendance was theoretically compulsory, students frequently skipped classes without a satisfactory excuse. They would explain an absence on the grounds of a personal illness or the illness or death of a parent. A student claiming illness had to be examined by Mueller or Hoffmann before his explanation was accepted.

Another Japanese practice Mueller could not abide was their prompt acceptance, *tadaima* (immediately), of an assigned task, and their subsequent failure to carry it out. Mueller scolded the students repeatedly for this behavior, and they eventually learned to respond promptly to his requests, which they referred to as *tadaima Germanica*. On the other hand, they continued to dawdle at a request from a Japanese—*tadaima Japonica*.

The students were required to wear a German-style uniform consisting of a close-fitting gray jacket and trousers, a blue cap, and leather boots; their hair had to be clipped in the German tradition to accommodate the cap. Whereas they had been accustomed to the traditional loose-fitting robes, they now went to the opposite extreme by having their uniforms tailored so tight that their movements were restricted and awkward. They also found the uniforms far too drab, so they had their jackets lined and collars trimmed with brightly hued violet, red, or blue silk.

The interpreters were required to wear European suits, and they found the change in attire even more difficult to cope with. It was an amusing

---

[34]Theodor Hoffmann, "Die Heilkunde in Japan und Japanische Aerzte," *Mitteilungen der deutschen Gesellschaft für Natur- und Völkerkunde Ostasiens,* 1873, *1:* 25.

sight when they struggled in and out of coat sleeves and trouser legs when they were used to slipping into a wide-sleeved flowing robe.

Mueller recalled one example of the problem in adjusting:

On New Year's Day 1874, I saw an official in the required European clothing returning from a ceremony at the court. As he was leaving the palace he discovered that it had been raining and the streets were sloppy. Without a moment's hesitation he took off his trousers and now proceeded along the street majestically attired in a black swallow-tail coat lined with white silk, a white vest, black top hat, holding an umbrella, wearing Japanese sandals, and covered below the waist by nothing more than a loincloth, which he wore only because of the threat of severe punishment.[35]

The study habits of Japanese students boasted none of the methodical steadfastness and punctuality characteristic of the Germans. This could be ascribed to the absence in Japan of a uniform system of keeping time. The day and the night were divided into six variable units called *toki* (parts), and the length of a *toki* not only changed every two weeks but also varied with the latitude and even within the limits of a large city. Thus in Tokyo on any one day, *toki* varied from one and a half to two and a half hours in different parts of the city. It was therefore almost impossible for a Japanese to adhere to a schedule. Mueller tolerated these irregularities for a few months and then required all students to purchase European watches and synchronize them to a uniform time schedule.

Another barrier to establishing an orderly teaching schedule was the fact that there was no week in the Japanese calendar. Instead, the first, seventh, thirteenth, nineteenth, and twenty-fifth days of each month were designated for rest. The problem was compounded by the occurrence of numerous and often unscheduled holidays; it was solved by introducing the European week.

On at least two occasions Mueller was vexed by what he termed "the unreliability of the Japanese . . . their desire to deceive foreigners and thereby deck themselves with foreign plumes." In 1874 the administration of the school told him that a large sum had been granted to establish a library. Mueller and the German staff held a number of meetings to prepare a list of books, but after many months of inaction recognized that the whole plan was a hoax. No funds were available, and the Japanese wanted the list solely for their own use at some future date. As another example of the Japanese unreliability, at the Centennial Exposition in Philadelphia in 1876, they exhibited as their own invention an ingenious bamboo stretcher in which the hollow interior of the bamboo poles could be used to store fluids and dressings. In actuality they had filched the plans from Mueller but had not informed him nor given him any credit.[36]

The successive frustrations at times drove Mueller to the verge of despair, but his spirits were restored by his fondness for the students and

[35]Mueller, "Tokio Igaku," p. 451.
[36]Ibid., pp. 452-53.

the esteem in which he was held: "Twice I was close to resigning, but the exceptionally talented students and the occasional recognition that I received gave me renewed incentives that, however, were soon dampened by new obstacles. I led a life of alternating hope and fear and anxiety."[37]

For a short time Mueller and Hoffmann and their wives had temporary quarters in the English hotel, the only foreign hostelry in Tokyo. They then moved into more permanent quarters in a main building of Kaneiji, the Buddhist family temple of the Tokugawa dynasty. Two Japanese youths lived with the two families in order to learn German. One was the son of Iwasa Jun and the other, of Shiba Ryokai, a chief physician at the school.

For the first year the Germans found themselves under round-the-clock surveillance by the Japanese. A bodyguard of eight police—four mounted and four on foot—accompanied them every time they left the temple compound, ostensibly to protect them but, more likely, in order to follow their movements. When the Germans passed through a *sekisho* separating one section of the city from another, their escorts handed the gatekeeper small wooden plates on which their names were stamped. All the plates were collected and rcorded with the name of the *sekisho* at the end of each day.

A doorkeeper at their residence recorded all arrivals and departures and the names of any guests. This information was also passed on daily to the police. These practices, so repugnant to the Germans, continued until the end of 1872, when after many complaints from Mueller the number of guards was reduced to four; the following year the practice was discontinued altogether.

Mueller's efforts to take lessons in Japanese from native instructors were another source of discomfiture. After one and a half years with a private tutor, he found the sentence structure too complex; and, with (typical) Japanese show of deference, his teacher was reluctant to correct any errors in his pronunciation. Furthermore, Mueller studied Japanese from a text written in the stilted style of archaic manuscripts, and his speech reflected this style. Thus, when he gave orders to the household servants in his antiquated and mispronounced Japanese, they fled to his wife, who spoke sufficient conversational Japanese to be able to communicate with them. Mueller eventually dismissed his tutor, and through his daily intercourse with the Japanese acquired enough fluency in the language and in the colloquial manner of expression to converse with patients and travel throughout the country with relative ease.

On the Kaiser's birthday, March 22, 1873, Ambassador Brandt and Mueller convened a small group of Germans residing in Yokohama and Tokyo to found a scientific and cultural society, the Deutsche Gesellschaft für Natur- und Völkerkunde Ostasiens. Their objective was "to create a common focal point for individual scientific endeavors and thereby en-

---

[37] Ibid., p. 326.

courage research on one hand, and on the other, to make available results of research to a wider audience."[38]

At its first general meeting on April 26 of that year, the group adopted statutes that included a statement that the society would afford its members opportunities for the exchange of views and experiences on East Asia and thereby promote investigations of the countries of the region. The society would also publish a journal, *Mitteilungen der deutschen Gesellschaft für Natur- und Völkerkunde Ostasiens,* for the dissemination of knowledge on East Asia.

The location of the monthly meetings would alternate between Tokyo and Yokohama. The language of the meetings and of the publication would be German, but the executive committee was empowered to grant the right to speak in another language to a member or a guest who had not mastered German. At no meeting, however, could more than one lecture be presented in another language.

Membership was not restricted to Germans, nor to residents of Japan. The international membership expanded as the society enrolled members in Hong Kong, Shanghai, Peking, Paris, and Berlin.

The first officers for 1873 were as follows: chairman, Ambassador Brandt; vice-chairman, Mueller; secretaries, Franz M. Hilgendorf of the premedical faculty and P. Kemperman, secretary-treasurer of the imperial German embassy; librarian, Cochius (also of the premedical faculty); and archivist, E. Mammelsdorff. Thus, three of the six founding officers were on the faculty of the medical school.

The papers presented at the meetings covered a broad range of fields: archeology, botany, meteorology, anthropology, geography, medicine, topography, Japanese culture, Japanese tea societies, Japanese skulls, Japanese history, *kakke* (beriberi), Mt. Fujiyama, equipment to be taken on an expedition to Hokkaido, and midwifery in Japan. Mueller demonstrated his versatility by presenting an extensive discourse on Japanese music and musical instruments.

The library of the society grew rapidly, and in his annual report of January 31, 1874, Brandt stated that it contained 273 volumes, of which half were in Japanese and half were foreign. The holdings included specimens from natural history and ethnography, as well as products of Japanese art and industry. Brandt presented a collection of lace from Ceylon. Other early donations included models of a Japanese teahouse and temple, samples of Japanese medicines, photographs of silk spinning and weaving, and the skeleton of an Ainu.

A major acquisition in the summer of 1873 was the library of Alexander von Siebold, an interpreter with the British legation, along with one of the collections of Japonica of his famous father, Philipp Franz Balthasar von Siebold, that the family had turned over to the government of Japan. Exchanges of *Metteilungen* with other journals were established, with a total of fifty-four far-flung scientific and cultural societies in such centers as Batavia, Berlin, Dresden, Vienna, Leipzig, Turin, the Smithsonian Institution (in Washington, D. C.), Amsterdam, and Moscow.

At a time when Britain, France, Russia, and Germany were at the height of their imperialistic ambitions in the Far East, Mueller recognized that the medical school was an important instrument for spreading German influence beyond the sphere of education:

The physicians and pharmacists who have been trained in German and will gradually spread across this empire could become our best pioneers for building strong relationships between our two countries. At first the Japanese purchased German texts, drugs, instruments, and chemicals from the medical school and the hospital. Later our products became available more widely, and the Japanese were completely satisfied with them. Therefore, they expanded business relationships with us, and an increasingly active trade was developed.[39]

Another testimonial to the broadening impact of the school had come from the *Zentralverein für Handelsgeographie* (Central Organization for International Trade), which on several occasions had acclaimed its positive role in the expansion of commerce with Germany.

In October 1874, Nagayo Sensai succeeded Sagara Chian as director of the school and of the medical bureau. Henceforth, Sagara's life went into a decline. His arrogant and abrasive manner intensified, and he antagonized so many people that he was friendless and soon destitute as well. For a brief period, Sagara was imprisoned, and he died in a situation of miserable squalor.

A member of the Omura family of medical men on Kyushu, Nagayo was one of Ogata Koan's leading pupils at Tekitekisai Juku. At Ogata's urging, in 1860 Nagayo enrolled as a student of Pompe van Meerdervoort. For Nagayo, it was a new world: "Dr. Matsumoto [Matsumoto Ryojun] introduced me to Dr. Pompe but I could not speak a word and just shook hands because he was the first foreigner I ever saw."[40]

Nagayo became the Japanese director of the Nagasaki school but was summoned to Tokyo for a governmental medical post soon after the restoration. He served as medical member of the Iwakura Tomomi mission to America and Europe in 1871-1873 and concentrated on medical and public-health programs in the United States, Britain, and Germany. As he recalled in his autobiographical *Shokoshishi*, "I became aware that there must be a special organization for the protection of all aspects of the health of the people." This would involve not only prevention of communicable diseases but also assistance to the poor and development of public sanitation.[41]

[39]Mueller, "Tokio Igaku," p. 449.
[40]Nagayo Sensai, *Shōkō Shishi* (Tokyo: Tohodo Shoten, 1900), p. 11.
[41]Quoted in F. Ohtani, *One Hundred Years of Health Progress in Japan* (Tokyo: International Medical Foundation of Japan, 1971), p. 16.

On the basis of his observations, Nagayo spent one year drafting *Isei* (medical system), which was promulgated in 1874. The essential features of *Isei* were as follows:

1. Division of the country into seven Health Districts controlled by the Medical Bureau in Tokyo. The districts were to be staffed by practitioners of medicine, pharmacists, and veterinarians, who in turn would regulate activities in their fields. Vital statistics, including births, communicable diseases, and mortality, would be recorded.

2. Medical schools to conduct a preparatory course of two years and a five-year medical currciculum. Regulations specified the location of the schools, patterns of staffing, and curriculum.

3. Licensing of medical graduates after two years of practical experience, with provisional licenses for those already in practice. Licensing for midwives and for practitioners of acupuncture and moxibustion as well was required.

4. Licensing and regulations for all hospitals.

5. A central bureau in Tokyo, with branch offices in the prefectures. Regulations were defined for licensing pharmacists and their assistants, as well as apprentices, and for the operation of pharmacies.

Such far-reaching a comprehensive reforms could not come about overnight, and in the eyes of some officials, Nagayo's program was too idealistic.

Hasegawa Yasushi, who had been a student supervisor when Mueller arrived in Japan, was temperamentally akin to Sagara Chian, for both were firebrands. Therefore, when *Mombusho* replaced Sagara, Hasegawa opposed the appointment vociferously. Since his relationships with *Mombusho* were already tenuous, the ministry now determined to remove him from Tokyo and urged Hasegawa to accept the appointment of *bucho* (dean) at Nagasaki Igakko. Just two weeks after he took up his new post at Nagasaki, on October 12, 1874, *Mombusho* decided to convert the hospital to military use for treating casualties of the war with Formosa. Hasegawa was compelled by *Mombusho* to relinquish his title and also forbidden to enter the premises of the medical school and the hospital. These moves infuriated him, and in a vengeful mood he cleaned out the library, laboratories, and cash box at Igakko in Nagasaki and took them to Tokyo.[42]

With the conversion of Yojosho in Nagasaki to a military hospital for casualties from the Formosan expedition, the students at Nagasaki were allowed to transfer to Tokyo Igakko. Since they were not prepared for the demanding curriculum and a teaching program in German, it was found necessary in May 1875 to establish a less demanding four-year program,

---

[42]Ogawa Teizo, ed., *Tokyo Daigaku Igakubu Hyakunenshi, 1858-1958* (Tokyo: Kinenkai, 1967), pp. 266-70). The Centenary History of Nagasaki Medicine (*Nagasaki Igaku Hyakunenshi*) cites another example of Hasegawa's petulance. Theodor H. Hoffmann was rather diffident and usually late for his lectures. Hasegawa is said to have stood by the portals with a lash, in a futile effort to intimidate him.

Igaku Tsugakusei Kyojo (medical study, commuting students). All of the teaching was in Japanese by junior staff members and by former students at Igakujo in the pre-German era. Other students were allowed to enroll in the program, which was always completely separate from the German curriculum and staff.

As August 1874 approached, and with it the expiration date of Mueller and Hoffmann's contracts, the Japanese asked the two men to continue their work under a new contract with *Mombusho*. They found this proposal completely unacceptable, however, and made plans to return to Europe. The officials then recognized that the services Mueller and Hoffmann were rendering would be indispensable until their successors arrived. Among their distinguished patients were Iwakura Tomomi (1825-1883), counselor and senior minister, and Kido Koin (1833-1871), also a high governmental official. Mueller and Hoffmann were therefore appointed personal physicians to the *Tenno,* which placed them in an independent position; they also continued to teach medicine.

At the end of 1874, Albrecht Ludwig Agathon Wernich (1843-1896) arrived to succeed Hoffmann, and Emil August Wilhelm Schultze (1840-1925) came from Berlin as Mueller's successor. Mueller and Hoffmann completed their duties at Igakujo by Easter 1875, and *Mombusho* gave a sumptuous banquet in their honor. It had a special significance in Japan because for the first time, the wives were allowed to attend. The German doctors then received the highest honor the Japanese could confer on them, the Order of the Rising Sun and the imperial brocades.

During the stewardship of Mueller and Hoffman, the status of the medical profession had risen dramatically. Young men from the most distinguished and wealthiest families were now enrolling at Igakujo, in contrast to the students of just four years earlier, who had come from the lower social and economic strata.

On the long homeward passage, Mueller recorded his experiences in Japan, but decided to defer publication for ten years. He did so to avoid disturbing the Japanese, "to whom I am obliged by so much friendliness and manifestations of recognition and love."[43]

Mueller was appointed director of the rehabilitation hospital in Berlin on his return to Germany and died after a long illness on October 13, 1893. His greatest accomplishment had been the establishment of the new school at a standard comparable to that of the better European medical institutions. Yet there was still much to be done. A complete faculty needed to be recruited, and a modern physical plant had to be erected. As the caliber of the students improved, they would expect more challenging lectures. The demands for consultations on private patients were growing steadily. These were the problems confronting the Germans who succeeded Mueller and Hoffmann, and their Japanese counterparts.

[43]Mueller, "Tokio Igaku," p. 315.

Wilhelm Schultze's son described him as being a very natural man who never strove for the limelight; he was somewhat antisocial and preferred a small group of close acquaintances to large gatherings. His candor verged on bluntness. Music was his favorite diversion, and he performed skillfully on the piano and the zither. Owing to his modesty and an overly critical attitude toward his own accomplishments, he failed to publish a single scholarly paper during his seven years in Japan.

Born at Spittelmacht in Berlin, March 28, 1849, the son of a textile merchant, Schultze established a brilliant record at Berlin's *Französisches Gymnasium,* one of the two leading *Gymnasia* in the city. He demonstrated a special fluency in French and English, and at commencement, April 13, 1859, was ranked *Primus omnium.* His primary interest was in science, especially chemistry and toxicology, but he entered medical studies because he was awarded a scholarship. He enrolled at the Faculty of Medicine, from which he graduated on July 18, 1863. After two years in compulsory military medical duty, Schultze served in the Seven Weeks' War. At the termination of the campaigns, he returned to the *Pépinière* to continue training in surgery. On November 7, 1868, he received the highest grade on the *Physikatsexamen* for a commission in the army sanitary corps.

At the outbreak of the Franco-Prussian War, Schultze joined the Prussian armies in the field, and when the siege of Paris began in the fall of 1870, he was posted to the First Field Hospital at Versailles. After the surrender of France on January 28, 1871, he returned to the *Pépinière* as captain, with a collateral appointment as chief librarian. In October, 1871, Schultze began a one-year study leave to investigate the treatment of war wounds in Holland and Britain. His period with Lord Lister was especially fruitful for he not only learned Lister's antiseptic techniques but also gained a degree of mastery of the English language.

On his return to Berlin, Schultze presented a major lecture on Listerian antisepsis before the Military Medical Society. This won him the post-humous epithet "Lister's apostle in Germany."[44] The publication of the lecture in *Clinical Lectures* contributed to the great enthusiasm with which Listerian antisepsis was adopted in Germany, in comparison with other countries in Europe and England.

During the next two years Schultze served with distinction as first assistant in the surgical clinic of Adolf Bardeleben at La Charité. This was a turning point in his career. When the search was underway for a successor to Mueller, it focussed on Berlin, and Schultze, as Bardeleben's first assistant, was the obvious candidate.

Theodor Hoffmann's successor, Albrecht Ludwig Agathon Wernich, and Schultze furnished a study in contrasts. While Schultze found it

---

[44]Geheimrat Bäumler, Obituary of Wilhelm Schultze, "Ein Pionier der Listerschen Wund-behandlung in Deutschland," *Münchner medizinische Wochenschrift,* 30 January 1925, *72:* 188.

impossible to produce scholarly essays, Wernich was, next to Erwin Baelz, his own successor, one of the most prolific writers at the Tokyo faculty.

Wernich studied medicine at the illustrious Faculty of Medicine at the University of Königsberg. During his student days, the leading member of the faculty was Friedrich Daniel von Recklinghausen (1833-1910), who held the chair in pathology for over thirty years and published important studies on the pathology of bone and multiple neurofibromatosis. After graduating in 1867, Wernich qualified in internal medicine at Berlin and then trained in obstetrics-gynecology. His studies for the *Habilitation* were interrupted by service in the Franco-Prussian War, but he completed his dissertation in 1874.

Wernich accepted an invitation from *Mombusho* soon after he completed the *Habilitation*. When he crossed the United States he was struck by the hostility he found manifested toward the Japanese: even among "miners and barkeepers."[45] This antipathy reminded him of reports from German *O-yatoi* who expressed a similar contempt. On the other hand, he was reassured by the appealing portrait that Ambassador Max von Brandt drew of life there, especially the high social status of the Germans.

Wernich wrote an extensive and illuminating commentary on the medical students. They had adjusted remarkably well in three years to the study of a totally new system of medicine, taught in an alien tongue by foreign professors and under a system of learning that was strange to them.

Their progress in mastering the German language was satisfactory, but Wernich found that their spoken German was "gruff, halting, and hesitant, much as we are accustomed to hear it spoken by a Russian." In his view, the Japanese had special talents in languages and were enthusiastic about learning the German alphabet. Their long training in writing Japanese characters gave them "great success in developing a clear and aesthetically pleasant penmanship." Since Japan had been sealed from the West for two centuries, they were especially keen on geography and made a hobby of drawing maps: "Many students became adept cartographers and maintained that interest despite the fact that they were almost always overburdened with work."[46]

Mathematics was a challenge: "At first all of the students, even the most talented, had difficulty with mathematics. The adult Japanese always perform the most simple numerical procedures of addition and subtraction on their adding machines [the Chinese abacus, known in Japan as the *soroban*]. Multiplying and dividing, which require a bit of memory and numerical knowledge acquired in early youth, were carried out slowly and awkwardly."[47]

---

[45] A. Wernich, "Über die Fortschritte der modernischen Medizin in Japan," *Berliner klinische Wochenschrift* 1975, *12*: 447.

[46] A. Wernich, "Zur Geschichte der Medizin in Japan." *Rohlf's Archiv für Geschichte der Medicin und medicinische Geographie*, 1878, *1*: 234.

[47] Ibid.

For the students, the courses in botany, chemistry, and zoology were also high points of the curriculum. All the Japanese seemed to understand physics instinctively.

Wernich was impressed to find that the best Tokyo students matched German students in their ability in the basic sciences: "It is by no means an exaggeration to say that in the early years of study, six of our best and most conscientious students would have competed on an equal basis with six medical students selected at random from any German university."[48]

In general, though, the Japanese by the time of graduation were no better than German country doctors who had completed training a number of decades earlier:

The best of the graduates are now approximately equal to our elderly rural physicians in regard to their skills, comprehension of their responsibilities, and especially their scientific background. Those who are less capable will never attain self-confidence or be able to develop any skills as rapidly as do even our lazy German students, who barely pass their examinations and then head for the country to open a rural practice.[49]

On the other hand, the commitment of the students to their studies was remarkable:

While we Germans are able to master profound questions with relative ease, it is only the strong determination of an East Asian as is so well demonstrated by our students that allows them to master the most elementary aspects of medical practice. . . . They work their way through a mass of knowledge and of technical skills with remarkable perseverance.[50]

Because the students in his first class were not sufficiently familiar with German, Wernich found it impossible to teach them the art of writing good medical histories. It was necessary to communicate with them through an interpreter, and he restricted his presentations to terse and superficial diagnoses:

However, the students in the second class, to whom I taught diagnostics and other methods of examining patients, were able to express themselves in correct and proper German as long as the discussions were on the subject matter, but they became withdrawn and upset when any new German expression was introduced. They viewed all complicated sentences with suspicion.[51]

The students' bedside manner was admirable: they showed "a great patience in observation, a certain reliability in carrying out a prescribed

[48] Ibid., p. 237.
[49] Ibid.
[50] Ibid., pp. 235-36.
[51] Ibid., p. 237.

course of treatment, gentleness, and dedication to the welfare of the patient.
. . . They avoid all gruffness, even toward the poor and uneducated
patients." However, the students made every effort to avoid poor patients
afflicted with the more dreadful diseases, such as leprosy.[52]

Wernich also appraised the state of medicine and its practitioners. The
physicians took special pride in exhibiting Western medical instruments:
"Practically every progressive doctor, even those in the hinterland, has
acquired a percussion hammer, a pleximeter, and probably even a medical
thermometer. He displays them in his belt with pride and for all to see."[53]
Yet the practitioners, in line with Japanese traditions, desired an arm's-
length relationship with their patients. Otherwise, they feared, they would
become enmeshed in a lifelong series of obligations involving the exchange
of gifts, adoptions, and welfare responsibilities.

So far, European medical science had had little influence in the
provinces, but European doctors scattered across the empire were respected
by the Japanese practitioners, who frequently sought them as consultants.
A clinical journal for practitioners published by the government presented
to its readership the most significant disease problems seen in the clinics of
Tokyo, along with illustrated descriptions of surgical operations. Written
exclusively in Japanese, it was sent to provincial governors for free distribution to their doctors. At the time of Wernich's departure in 1876, sixteen
volumes had appeared at irregular intervals.

The Education Law of 1872 established compulsory elementary education as a prerequisite for success in all occupations and professions. It
made primary education available to girls and boys of all social classes,
with an opportunity for the more talented to go on to advanced studies.
During his two years in Japan, Wernich concluded that a sound start had
been made on implementing this law: "Even the smallest villages have
elementary schools—usually a very ordinary room in a tiny house, in which
there are several groups of twenty students."[54] Although these houses had
not been erected as schools, they were readily identified as such:

The exterior is easily recognized by the large number of children's shoes deposited
before the entrance. . . . One can tell it is a school when one is a block away by the
loud, shrill voices of the children repeating gleefully and persistently the syllabus,
which is recited by the teacher in a deep voice, and whoever is still in doubt has
only to wait until the crowd of children, who have been confined for such a long
period, streams through the narrow doorway, swinging their few school materials in
black bags. Happily and with lightninglike swiftness, they slip into their wooden
shoes.[55]

[52] Ibid.
[53] Ibid., pp. 237-38.
[54] A. Wernich, "Über Ausbreitung und Bedeutung der neuen Culturbestrebungen in
Japan," *Deutsche Zeit- und Streitfragen*, 1877, *6*(93): 485.
[55] Ibid., pp. 485-86.

As it had done for centuries, instruction in writing turned upon the syllabic system of *katakana* with its large characters drawn with a brush and India ink. The children were required to memorize by constant repetition.

While both boys and girls had the same learning experience in primary school, most girls in rural schools were then diverted to an inferior program. They continued to learn only *katakana,* while the boys were advanced to the more scholarly and useful cursive writing of *hiragana* as well as to Chinese characters. Such discrimination made it impossible for women to read the newspapers, all of which were published in *hiragana.*

Fortunately, the empress was pressing for the beginning of suffrage, and the first newspaper in *katakana* had just been published. Her efforts to establish special *jyokoba* (female schools) met with a significant degree of success. The empress enhanced the prestige of the program by making personal visits to the schools.

The enthusiasm for female education even penetrated the world of the geisha, as a newspaper reported in the summer of 1876: "According to rumors, the singing girls and other women of doubtful repute from the Nagasaki department have petitioned the government for permission to construct a school at their own expense and to open it as soon as possible."[56]

Wernich became hypercritical of the Japanese and their country. He bored his German colleagues with his tirades and grew increasingly disenchanted with his position. He left Japan in December 1876 for a career as a governmental doctor. He prepared monographs on medical history, epidemics, and hygiene and carried out research in epidemiology and communicable diseases.

[56] Ibid., pp. 483-84.

6

Erwin Baelz

The German professor Erwin Baelz, who succeeded Wernich, was the foremost physician in Meiji Japan. He was a gifted and compassionate doctor whose prestigious practice included the imperial family and leading governmental dignitaries. Baelz's range of scholarship spanned tropical and nutritional diseases, neuropsychiatric disorders, physical anthropology, and balneotherapy. In all of these fields he was both a thoughtful and a prolific writer.

Baelz was a Swabian, born at Bietigheim, near Stuttgart, on January 13, 1849. At the age of five, he entered the Bietigheim *Volksschule* and after three years advanced to the local Latin school. He then studied the classics and the sciences at the Eberhard-Ludwigs-Gymnasium in Stuttgart and demonstrated particular aptitude in the natural sciences, French, and Latin. In his leisure hours he frequently read books on world geography and studied maps.

Having achieved high grades on the final examination at the *Gymnasium,* Baelz enrolled in 1866 at Tuebingen, the university of his native *Land.* Professor Felix Hoppe-Selyer (1825-1895), a pioneer in physiological chemistry, was the most distinguished member of its faculty. Another faculty member, Karl Vierordt (1818-1884), the professor of physiology, was the inventor of the sphygmograph.

Baelz enjoyed a close friendship with a classmate, Robert Wiedersheim, later professor of anatomy at Freiburg and the author of a book on the comparative anatomy of vertebrates. Another friend of his at Tuebingen, Hermann Fehling (1847-1925), developed the quantitative test that bears his name for sugar in the urine. Baelz was also an enthusiastic participant in the Germania Students Association, one of the oldest student unions in Germany; the Germania Association at that time was devoting its youthful vigor to support of Bismarck's drive to unite Germany.

At the end of his basic-science studies, Baelz followed the style of most German medical students by moving on to another faculty. He selected the University of Leipzig primarily because of the luster of his Swabian compatriot there, Professor Karl Reinhold August W. Wunderlich (1815-1877), Germany's most popular teacher of internal medicine. Wunderlich's approach to medicine had a profound influence on Baelz and on his subsequent career. He, too, had studied at Tuebingen but interrupted his time there to spend one year observing practical clinical medicine in Paris. He returned to Tuebingen and earned his *Habilitation* in the spring of 1840. At that time, Paris and Vienna, with their diametrically opposed approaches to medical education, were the major influences on the German schools, and Wunderlich spent several months in the autumn of 1840 at the Vienna civic hospital. The following year, his observations were published at Stuttgart under the title *Vienna and Paris.* Wunderlich pointed out that while Vienna strongly emphasized therapeutic nihilism, Paris medicine was based on careful clinical studies of patients. In contrast to the nihilistic attitude of the Viennese, the French advocated active therapeusis. By following the Paris model, Wunderlich attained great popularity both as a teacher and as a practitioner.

Karl Wunderlich's most outstanding medical contribution came in 1868, when he founded clinical thermometry by publishing, after twenty years of recording patients' temperatures, his classic treatise *Das Verhalten der Eigenwärme in Krankheiten.*[1] The practical application of Wunderlich's treatise was made possible by Sir Thomas Clifford Allbutt (1836-1925), who devised the prototype of the modern clinical thermometer in 1867.

The general mobilization for the Franco-Prussian War in 1870 found Erwin Baelz serving as a surgeon's assistant with the Wuerttemburg troops. He helped to manage a severe dysentery epidemic near Sedan and, when peace was restored, returned to the study of medicine at Leipzig, where he graduated *summa cum laude,* April 18, 1872. Baelz then became an assistant in the Pathological Anatomy Institute at Leipzig and successfully defended his doctoral thesis on progressive bulbar paralysis.

The ensuing four years were pivotal in the development of Erwin Baelz's qualities as a physician. As first assistant to Wunderlich, he soon became imbued with the latter's clinical skills as well as with his humanitarianism and deep concern for the welfare of patients. And as Wunderlich became terminally ill with lymphosarcoma and miliary tuberculosis, Baelz took over his lectures to the medical students. His presentations were lucid and learned, and attracted even larger numbers of students than had those of his chief. With such a background, Baelz had every prospect of a fine academic career in Germany. At this point, he quite unexpectedly chose to go to Japan.

Baelz's decision to join the Faculty of Medicine at Tokyo is related to his contact with a Japanese patient at Leipzig. His son, Toku, explains in his introduction to his father's diary: "In the year 1875, a Japanese official came under his care. In the course of the treatment Baelz showed his interest in the patient's native country and was thereupon asked whether he would not like to get a firsthand knowledge of Japan."[2] Baelz replied

---

[1] Leipzig, 1868. See also K. A. Wunderlich, *Medical Thermometry,* 2nd ed., trans. W.B. Woodman (London: New Sydenham Society, 1871).

[2] Erwin Baelz, *Awakening Japan: The Diary of a German Doctor,* ed. by Toku Baelz, trans. by Eden and Cedar Paul (New York: Viking Press, 1932), pp. 3-4. The identity of the

immediately in the affirmative. In his diary he explained his decision: "Beyond question, I am leaving the safe soil of my homeland, and assured prospect, to confront an unknown destiny. . . . Eventful possibilities loom before me, and the gratification of an earnest wish. I, too, am to play a part in the diffusion of Western civilization among a gifted population eager for knowledge." On New Year's Eve, 1875, the Japanese Ministry in Berlin informed him that the terms he had proposed were acceptable, and on January 3, 1876, Baelz signed a two-year contract in Berlin in the presence of the Japanese minister, Aoki Shuzo. His appointment as professor of physiology and internal medicine included free voyage to Japan and return to Germany, free quarters, a salary of 16,200 German Marks per year payable monthly, and the privilege of holding a private practice.[3]

Minister Aoki Shuzo (1844-1914) became a close Japanese friend of the German medical mission, both in Germany and in Japan. (His association with medicine and medical men could be traced to his grandfather, Aoki Shusuke (1803-1863), who in September 1849 had assisted in the dissemination of cowpox vaccination soon after its introduction by Mohnike.)[4] Aoki Shuzo, born Miura Shuzo, was a son of the Miura family of Choshu. He was a talented student, and the clan sent him to Germany in 1868 to study international politics and the law. In 1874, he was appointed minister to Germany. In this ambassadorial position, he was the key Japanese in the recruitment of professors for the medical school. When he returned to Tokyo he became vice-minister of foreign affairs and was a frequent visitor to the homes of the professors in Kaga, in turn entertaining them in his residence.[5]

After Baelz arrived at Yokohama on June 8, 1876, his first medical-school contact was with Wernich, who was now outspoken in his antipathy toward the Japanese. He described them to Baelz as "utterly decayed and neurotic. . . . there are really no healthy Japanese left."[6]

As early as May 1870, Sagara Chian proposed that the medical school and hospital should move from the low-lying, damp, humid Todo *yashiki.* He suggested a site in Ueno Park, but Antonius Bauduin, who was serving as an interim teacher at Igakujo, urged that the new site should be the Kaga *yashiki,* located in the higher and drier Hongo section near Ueno Park. In October 1874 the decision was made to build a new facility at the

official is unclear; two Japanese medical historians speculate that the Japanese was Sagara Gentei (or Motosada), a younger brother of Sagara Chian. Ishibashi Chosei and Ogawa Teizo, *O-yatoi Gaikokujin-Igaku* (Tokyo: Kajima Kenkyusho Shuppankai, 1969), pp. 110-11.

[3] Baelz, *Awakening Japan,* p. 4.

[4] *Encyclopedia Japonica,* vol. I (Shokakukan: November 20, 1967).

[5] In a letter to Berlin of September 19, 1879, Emma Schultze, wife of the professor of surgery, tells of sitting with Aoki during a formal celebration. He had accompanied the Schultzes to the ball, and Aoki was, she wrote, "so European and 'Berlinish' that one completely forgets that dear Aoki is a Japanese, and I feel completely at home."

[6] Baelz, *Awakening Japan,* p. 25.

yashiki. Construction of the hospital and main building of the medical school began in July 1875, and the faculty occupied their new quarters during November-December 1876. Meanwhile the faculty families had moved from the old temples of Ueno to the *yashiki.*

The grounds of the *yashiki* had been given to Maeda Toshitsune, *daimyo* of the Kaga clan, by Tokugawa Ieyasu (1542-1616). The gift was a reward for Maeda's military support of the Tokugawa when they laid siege to Osaka Castle in 1614-1615 in order to destroy their main enemy, Toyotomi Hideyori.[7] A ceremonial red gate, Akamon, was built when in 1827 the thirteen-year-old Nariyasu, hereditary leader of the Maeda family, who were the *daimyo* of Kaga, was to be married to Yohime, daughter of the shogun Tokugawa Ienari. Tradition required that a *daimyo* whose family was marrying to the Tokugawa erect a spacious home with a red gate, through which the bride and the wedding procession entered.

After the Meiji restoration, the Maeda family were allowed to maintain their residence at the *yashiki.* The red gate became the entrance of Tokyo University in 1903, and since then the university has been popularly referred to as Akamon. The gate withstood the 1923 earthquake that destroyed much of Tokyo; on December 14, 1931, Akamon was designated a national treasure. It subsequently survived the bombings and fires of World War II and was repaired in 1961.

Franz M. Hilgendorf, who was returning to Germany with a comprehensive collection of marine specimens, invited Baelz to share his quarters at the *yashiki* until his ship sailed. Of the six German residences, it was the most attractive. The house was situated at the summit of a hill, and Baelz found the view overlooking the park charming. But his chief delight was the hitherto neglected garden, and soon he had Japanese gardeners restoring it and planting flowers, shrubbery, and trees. The cultivation of *bonsai* (dwarf trees) and the art of flower arranging (*ikebana*) became two of Baelz's principal hobbies, and during the warm months the homes at the *yashiki* were fragrant with his blossoms. In 1879 his colleagues allowed him to restore the spacious garden that had belonged to the *daimyo* of the Kaga fief.[8]

One month after his arrival, Baelz made the first of his many explorations of the interior of the country in order to study topography, the people and their customs, and balneology. He also began to collect specimens of Japanese art; varieties of the old-fashioned, long, curved sword with blades equal to the finest from Damascus; and daggers for the ritual *seppuku.*

Baelz was appalled by the medical school's temporary facilities, "a hideous old barrack of a place, a low wooden shedlike structure with

[7] Ogawa Teizo, ed., *Tokyo Daigaku Igakubu Hyakunenshi, 1858-1958.* Tokyo Daigaku Igakubu Soritsu Hyakunen Kinenkai (Tokyo, 1968), pp. 645-50.

[8] The lord of Kaga in Ishikawa on the Japan Sea was one of the wealthiest *daimyo,* with his four *yashiki* occupying over 250 acres and with staffs totalling several thousand. The *yashiki* in which Baelz and other members of the medical mission resided was renowned for its beautiful gardens.

sliding doors."[9] The inner grounds displayed about the same degree of cleanliness as a pig sty. But he took heart when he learned that a new physical plant would be completed by the end of the year.

Just two days after he arrived, Baelz gave his first lecture in physiology and materia medica. The students' understanding of the German language had improved to such a point that they seldom needed an interpreter; Baelz was impressed. On the examination in histology most of the students ranked in the upper bracket.

Most of November was spent in moving to the new facilities, and on December 6, 1876, the new hospital opened. Ernest Tiegel, newly arrived from Germany, took over the teaching of physiology, and Baelz was happy that he could devote his entire time to clinical medicine.

With the opening of the hospital, the opportunities for private practice increased, and the money and expensive gifts to be derived from it made the clinical professors' posts particularly attractive. The doctors observed the Japanese custom of neither submitting a bill nor handling money directly. The decorous envelope with the special red band that denoted a gift was deposited in the professor's office. Frequently a woodblock print, a piece of lacquer ware, pottery, a painted scroll, or some other gift would be added.

The physicians placed their substantial earnings in the German savings bank at Yokohama and also forwarded them to accounts in Germany. Baelz's practice was so lucrative that he was able to purchase property, most of it near spas, so that he could pursue his interest in balneotherapy. He was also able to acquire a country residence and a summer home on the lower slopes of Fujiyama.

On January 13, 1878, Wilhelm Schultze, the professor of surgery, returned to Berlin on home leave; he hoped to find a wife soon. Within a few weeks he met Emma Wegscheider, the daughter of a distinguished *Geheimrat* German physician. In a whirlwind courtship, they were betrothed on March 6, 1878, and the marriage took place on April 25. When he and Emma were expecting their first child, Schultze recalled to her parents the considerable difference in their ages: "I shall never forget my debt that I was able to change from being an old, lonely bachelor to having a young wife with a happy family."[10] He assured Dr. and Mrs. Wegscheider that he was well aware of the sacrifice that they had made in entrusting young Emma to a husband about whom they knew so little, aware that they would be so far away for such a long time.

Emma was devoted to her husband and children and to making a comfortable home for them. She shared her husband's predilection for the simple social life of many German people in Japan. Through a stream of letters she maintained intimate ties with her family in Berlin. Although

[9] Baelz, *Awakening Japan*, p. 14.

[10] Letter, September 18, 1878. The letters and illustrative materials, as well as other sources on Schultze, were given to me by his granddaughter, Dr. Toska Hesekiel.

she was surrounded by physicians, Emma continued to seek the advice of her father on the health and rearing of their two children, Elisabeth (Lieschen), born January 15, 1879, and a son, Walter Hans, born June 15, 1880. Both children were delivered at home by the father, with Erwin Baelz assisting.

No sooner were they settled in their home than they installed a complete set of meteorological instruments for measuring temperature, direction and velocity of wind, rainfall, and barometric pressure. Recording their readings three times daily was one of Emma's responsibilities. Her morning hours were divided among spending one hour each on letter writing, playing the piano, and simultaneously practicing Japanese and sewing.

Emma's closest acquaintance was a distant relative, Clara (Klaerchen) Mayet, whose husband, Paul, beginning in 1875 was the principal economic adviser to the Japanese government. He dealt with a wide variety of fields, including agriculture, postal-savings institutions, insurance, and holidays. Klaerchen and Emma played piano duets every other day, and Emma accompanied Klaerchen's solos and vocal exercises. But Emma was repeatedly distressed by Klaerchen's "bold" appearance at parties in daring décolleté evening dresses. These were at odds with Emma's conservative style, and in her letters to Berlin she often expressed her dismay. She reported that at one gala event, Klaerchen had gone to the extreme of wearing a beauty spot.

The German colony in Tokyo numbered about forty, including the staff at the legation. Since several Germans took Japanese wives, the Japanese women in the community at times outnumbered the German wives. The Japanese wives, by contrast with the German ones, lavished their men with every attention. As one member of the German community confessed, "We must admit that these Japanese women cared for their German *dannasan* [masters] in the most selfless manner."[11]

At one end of the *yashiki* rose a steep hill; at its foot was the large Shinobazu pond, whose waters were covered with a myriad of lotuses. Beside the pond stood a charming red temple. Meticulously designed garden plots with stately ancient trees and flowering fruit bushes made the summer months especially pleasing to the eye.

As was true of other foreign nationals, the Germans' contacts with the Japanese were largely limited to those Japanese who could speak German. Wilhelm Schultze described the efforts of his countrymen to speak the natives' tongue as *verstummeltes Japanisch* (mutilated Japanese). In this isolated situation, the wives concentrated on their families and their friends at the *yashiki.* Emma noted one byproduct of this circumstance when she wrote, explaining to her mother that she was pregnant for a second time, that all but two of the wives living in the compound were in the same condition: "Among European ladies a most unusual fertility seems to reign";

[11]Kurt Meissner, *Deutsches in Japan, 1639-1939* (Stuttgart and Berlin: Deutsche Verlags-Anstalt, 1940), p. 67.

indeed, "There is a veritable treasure house of babies among the German wives."[12]

Frequent shipments from home provided the Germans with tinned and smoked foodstuffs, clothes, toys for the children, sheet music, and cigars for the husbands. Eagerly awaited letters, newspapers, and other publications arrived in batches; the families shared the papers. Correspondents in Germany were urged to use the Atlantic-Pacific mails rather than the slower routes through the Suez. Music was a favorite diversion: the families played solos and duets at home, and larger musical groups performed the chamber works of Bach, Beethoven, Haydn, Mozart, and Schubert.

The families depended on clothes from home to such a degree that when a Mrs. Naumann's baby was born one month premature, the other wives donated garments for the infant because the mother's box had not arrived. Mrs. Schultze had difficulty finding a satisfactory Japanese seamstress and was forced to drape her daughter, Lieschen, in Japanese costume when they left the *yashiki*. Japanese milk was unsatisfactory for human use, and so the Germans used condensed milk from America or Switzerland.

With Japanese servants constantly in attendance, chattering incessantly, the children soon became more fluent in Japanese than in their mother tongue. The servants also spoiled them dreadfully. The wealthier foreign families therefore preferred Chinese servants, partly because they were stricter with the children.

The servants were almost equally solicitous of Emma as of the children. When she practiced the piano in the summer, a servant would appear silently behind her with a fan. If she performed any household task, "they express their gratitude by bowing to the ground as though I had demonstrated the deepest love for them."[13] The servants believed that the Wegscheiders in Germany were wealthy *daimyo* because of the crates filled with gifts that they sent to Emma and Wilhelm.

The families celebrated Christmas in the Germanic tradition—the tables piled high with gifts from home and from friends in Japan. Emma would already have shipped a chest of Christmas gifts to Germany in mid-October. A Christmas tree decorated with candles in many colors and with Japanese sugar candy reached to the ceiling. Baelz, the Schultzes' closest friend, was their guest for Christmas dinner. Emma once gave him a foot muff that she had knitted with his initials on it, a jar of sour pickles, and a plate of Christmas cookies. But, in the Japanese tradition, Baelz was never accompanied on social occasions by his wife, Hana.[14]

Baelz's garden in the summer was luxuriant with beautiful blossoms from flowering-cherry, magnolia, peach, and quince trees. From this

---

[12] Letter, September 11, 1879. Emma Schultze's letters have been translated by Mrs. Charlotte Marshall.

[13] Letter, October 6, 1878.

[14] Arai Hatsu (who later changed her name to "Hana") was born on February 20, 1864, the daughter of a Tokyo shopkeeper. There are several different accounts of her relation-

copious supply, Baelz bedecked the Schultzes' home, from the first flowers of springtime until the end of autumn.

Emma especially enjoyed sightseeing in the vicinity of the *yashiki.* The conveyance was instantly available: "Clap hands or ring a bell and just call *jinrikisha* and two minutes later, the vehicle is awaiting us at the door." In the course of her frequent two-hour rides in the daytime and strolls in the evening, she found that the street scenes were "quaint and entertaining during the day, but the evenings are ten times more beautiful and interesting." At twilight, the narrow streets were illuminated with lanterns and torches carried by pedestrians: "a sea of red and white lanterns."

The street scenes were so different and diverting that Emma wished she had ten eyes instead of two:

The two most colorful shops were those with children's toys, and prettiest of all, those of the fruit dealers, who were especially skillful in arranging their fruit among layers of green leaves. The least attractive, because of their odor, are the shops in which every species of fish is sold; at low tables or on the ground old women roast and fry all sorts of Japanese goods on a *hibachi.* . . . One delights in seeing the high wooden shoes, the tiny pigtails of the men, the upswept hairstyle and the makeup of the women, and especially the policemen and soldiers in uniform, who have the appearance of our schoolboy in athletic costumes.

But she preferred the tranquility of their compound to the shouts of the hawkers and the chatter of pedestrians on the streets: "Here in our quiet Kaga *yashiki* we are spared all this."[15]

The Schultzes became accustomed to the frequent minor tremors that shook their house. However, one major quake in the early-morning hours created pandemonium, and many of the wives began preparing to leave the country.

The visit of Prince Heinrich, son of the Kaiser in 1879 was a social highlight. He was entertained luxuriously by the Japanese, who opened a

---

ship with Erwin Baelz. One (in *Tokyo Ijishinsi,* 1936) dates it to 1881, when she helped Baelz during a cholera epidemic. Another (in Felix Schottlender, *Erwin von Baelz*) places it in 1888, two years after Baelz returned from a trip to Germany. A third, and probably the most accurate, written by one of Hana's relatives (in *Meidai Igakubu Gakuyujiho,* December 1961), tells how a high-ranking official's wife saw Hana while the latter was working as a hairdresser or waitress; the woman recommended her as a member of Baelz's household staff in 1881. The census register reports their legal marriage as having taken place on November 28, 1904—after they had lived together as devoted husband and wife for twenty-three years.

After Baelz's death, Hana remained in Stuttgart while their only son, Toku, served in the war; she cared for Baelz's aged mother and his sister and wrote a book of memoirs, *Oshiutaisen toji no Doitsu,* which was published in 1933. She returned to Japan in 1922 with the hope of reclaiming Baelz's savings, but the Japanese government had seized them as property of the enemy during World War I. When Hana became ill, Dr. Scriba's son, Emil, and his wife took her into their home. She died of a stomach cancer in February 1937 and is buried in Stuttgart. See Ume Kajima, "Baelz Hana," *Erwin von Baelz Fujin no Shogai* (Tokyo: Kajima Shuppankai), 1977).

[15] Letter, October 6, 1878.

charming palace with a beautiful garden by the sea to serve as his residence. They supplied numerous cooks, servants, carriages, and horses and stationed a guard of honor in front of the palace. The prince presented the Order of the Black Eagle to the emperor. Emma feared that they had overwhelmed the lad with their characteristic hospitality: "The Japanese are known to be very hospitable and friendly to such guests. They dragged him from banquet to banquet, showed him all the sights: parades, festival performances in the theater, races, artists, etc."[16]

The German community held a splendid reception for the prince. Its main attraction was a Japanese acrobat climbing a ladder whose steps were made of sword blades; he performed a series of juggling and balancing acts. Across the lake of the *yashiki* floated some fifteen hundred multicolored illuminated balloons, and a grandiose fireworks display climaxed the festivities. After the prince departed, the entire German community signed a congratulatory card with felicitations to the Kaiser in honor of his fiftieth wedding anniversary.

The arrival of Adolf Erik von Nordenskold (1832-1901) at Yokohama on September 2, 1879, after he opened the Northeast Passage, occasioned another festive celebration.[17] In recognition of his feat, the English and the German East Asian Societies and the Asiatic Society of Japan joined in sponsoring a banquet at the largest hall in Tokyo. The Japanese marine band played during dinner and for dancing; Emma reported to her parents that it "played excellently since it has acquired a German conductor."[18]

The emperor's birthday party was the crowning annual social event for the Japanese. It was attended by representatives of all the nations that had missions in Japan. Emma, in her usual frugal manner, remodeled her conservative wedding gown, her only formal dress, by adding pink silk fringes. She was shocked when the daughter of the American ambassador, Judge John Bingham, waltzed by in a low-cut sleeveless dress and "very heavy makeup." Because of their craze for a Western life-style, the Japanese men dressed in formal European evening attire, while their wives were gowned in a combination of European and Japanese designs. The Chinese guests preferred their traditional raiments and radiated amiability: "The most amusing sight was the Chinese minister in his native costume. . . . He was elderly, smiled at every lady and shook her hand. The members of his entourage were also dressed in Chinese gowns."[19] Emma found the emperor's birthday party "far more sparkling than the festival for General Grant, which was dominated by Americans."[20]

---

[16]Letter, June 7, 1879.

[17]The Swedish Arctic explorer and geologist had sailed from Goteborg on the *Vega,* June 5, 1878, and rounded Cape Chelyuskin, Siberia. His ship was frozen in for the fall and winter west of the entrance to the Bering Strait and did not reach the Bering Sea until July 20, 1879.

[18]Letter, September 19, 1879.

[19]November 11, 1879.

[20]Letter, November 11, 1879. After he left the White House in 1877, General and Mrs. Grant began a round-the-world tour that lasted two and a half years. Japan was the last

In January 1880 Wilhelm and Emma visited Kyoto, where two Germans, Wagner in physics and chemistry and Scheube in medicine, were serving as teachers. Their excursion to descend the Hozu River rapids was a high point of the visit. They rode up the Arashiyama (storm mountain): "Wilhelm and I traveled in a carriage pulled by three men. Wagner with his lapdog rode in another pulled by two men, and Katzu, our servant, followed in a *jinrikisha.*" They took lunch on a little hill near a temple and then made the rugged ride down the Hozu River rapids: "one and a half hours through thirty-two small rapids. The river, with many bends, coursed between two steep mountain walls."[21]

On the same trip, the Schultzes hiked across Mount Hiei through the snows to Lake Biwa, the largest lake in Japan, and Emma compared the view to one in Switzerland: "the most beautiful aspect of the Lake of Geneva with the Dents du Midi."[22]

The Germans followed the "akademisch" style of the fatherland by taking long, secluded vacations. In the summer of 1880, the Schultzes spent two months at Nikko, which because of its beauty and high altitude was a favorite summer resort for Europeans. They sent their extensive provisions ahead in *jinrikishas* and included "two cases of canned milk; one case of beer and wine; two cases of vegetables, meat, and canned soups; a small case of sweetened lemonade, in cans; a large basket of ham, coffee, sugar, and flour; and finally, an old easy chair."[23]

They left the *yashiki* at dawn and traveled in a carriage drawn by a team that was changed every hour. At dusk they took a room in a *ryokan* (inn) that was infested with fleas, and left early the next day in *jinrikishas.* Emma was amazed at the strength of the men who pulled their conveyances up the mountainside to their homes, located at an altitude of 2,000 feet. They had rented their summer residence from a Buddhist priest, and it was charming—in the center of a vast garden that abounded with fruit trees, and overlooking a lake dotted with many small islands connected by arching bridges. On rainy days in June, the Schultzes studied a book on chess, and Wilhelm gave Emma lessons in elementary physics. She spent a major share of her time teaching discipline to Lieschen, who was stubborn and spoiled by her Japanese nurse. But most of the days were sunny, and the Schultzes took long walks on which they could enjoy the magnificent mountain scenery with its rivers, cascades, and stunning waterfalls.

His dedication to his position in the medical school bound Schultze to long working hours. He arrived at the hospital at eight in the morning with

---

country they visited, June through September 1879; the party to which Emma refers took place on August 25 at Ueno Park. Grant received a warm welcome in Japan, where the political leaders asked his advice on the value of representative institutions. He recommended caution in adopting them.

[21] Letter, January 19, 1880.
[22] Letter, January 30, 1880.
[23] Letter, July 24, 1880.

a full schedule in the surgical theater, lectures, and clinics, which occupied him until at least one in the afternoon. After an interval for dinner, he spent his afternoons with his students and private patients and visitors. He frequently worked at his desk at home until midnight, preparing for his tasks on the following day. Thus, he allowed himself little if any time for scholarly pursuit.

However, Schultze's total commitment to his tasks at the medical school drew official commendation. On December 25, 1875, he received a laudatory letter from Tanaka Fujimaro, vice-minister of education: "The students are making good progress because of your unflagging dedication; we appreciate your cordial care of the sick; and we express special gratitude to you for your major contributions in organizing the teaching program."[24]

At the time of his departure from Japan, Schultze enjoyed a variety of recognitions. A letter from Aoki Shuzo praised him as the "first to introduce antiseptic surgery to Japan," and went on: "Through the performance of many difficult operations such as ovariectomy and others, you have demonstrated your unique talents, as well as advancing European medical science in the most illustrious manner. We wish you every success in the future."[25]

A letter from former ambassador Von Eisendecher on January 20, 1883, was equally laudatory: "The undersigned, who was the imperial ambassador in Japan for seven years, 1875 to 1883, wishes to take this opportunity to express to his friend Schultze, major, medical corps, who was employed by the Japanese government as professor of surgery and ophthalmology during the same period, his profound gratitude for the major contributions of Dr. Schultze, which were recognized by everyone and were as well in the best interests of Germany."[26]

On the basis of strong recommendations from Bardeleben and Volkmann, his professors at Berlin, Schultze was appointed director and chief medical officer of the governmental hospital at Stettin. After six years his blunt candor cost him the post: when Princess Fredericka made an official visit to the hospital, Schultze went to great lengths to point out to her how many things, in his opinion, were inadequate at the institution.

The first Japanese graduates to go to Germany trained in the basic sciences: anatomy, physiology, and pathology. In the meantime, strong teaching programs were being developed by the German professors, but their research endeavors were hampered by a lack of laboratories and equipment. This was a factor that prompted most of them to return to Germany after short tenures at the school, by contrast with the extended stays of the clinical leaders. The first Japanese, Osawa Kenji, Miyake Hiizu, and Koganei Ryosei, who returned to professorships in the basic sciences, were a triumvirate that led the transition of the school over a period of twenty-five years to becoming an institution staffed exclusively by Japanese.

[24]Letter, December 25, 1875.
[25]Letter from Aoki Shuzo, January 20, 1883.
[26]Letter from Von Eisendecher, imperial minister, January 20, 1883.

The first dissection was performed at Igakujo on October 27, 1870, by Hasegawa Yasushi and Ishiguro Tadanori, after they had gained permission from a magistrate. They are said to have performed fifty-two dissections in the Kendo (Japanese fencing) Hall of the Todo *yashiki* in the ensuing two months.[27]

When Mueller began to teach anatomy, he appointed Taguchi Kazuyoshi as his assistant. Taguchi had been a *Rangakusha* in his youth and joined the staff at Toko at the beginning of the Meiji era. As his teaching text Mueller used a Dutch version of the *Anatomical Atlas* of Karl Heitzman (1836-1896), a favorite text in the German universities. It had been modified from the Dutch by Pompe van Meerdervoort for use by Japanese students.

The first European basic-science teacher, Friedrich Wilhelm Donitz (1833-1912), joined the faculty on July 18, 1873, and took over Mueller's responsibilities in anatomy. He had been recruited by Nagayo Sensai while Nagayo was in Germany with the Iwakura mission. Donitz had studied medicine in Berlin and trained in anatomy with Reichert and Frerichs. In Tokyo, he taught comparative anatomy, embryology, and gross anatomy. In 1876, Donitz was involved in a dispute with the Japanese authorities; considerable bitterness arose, and he left the school to teach in a clan school at Saga in Kyushu.

Wilhelm Schultze taught anatomy until the arrival of Hans Paul Bernhard Gierke (1847-1886), who had graduated from the medical faculty in Würzburg in 1872. After postgraduate studies on respiration at the physiology institute in Breslau, Gierke returned to Würzburg as prosector in anatomy and histology with Albrecht von Kolliker (1817-1907), a pioneer in cellular histology. On Kolliker's recommendation, Gierke was appointed to teach at Tokyo in 1876. Gierke was sick in mind and body, and he was forced to return to Breslau in May 1880; there he spent his final months in a mental hospital. He was an avid collector of ethnological specimens; at his death, his Japanese collection was purchased by the Prussian government.

Joseph Disse (1852-1912), successor to Gierke, graduated at Erlangen and studied with Wilhelm Waldeyer at Strassburg. He taught at Tokyo for seven years.

When Koganei Ryosei (or Yoshikiyo) completed postgraduate studies at Berlin in anatomy and histology, his research was with Waldeyer on the detailed structure of the iris. When he returned from Berlin in 1885, he became head of the Anatomy Institute. In May of that year, Taguchi Kazuyoshi, who had been on the staff of the Anatomy Institute for one decade, left for Berlin, where he spent two years in research under Wilhelm Waldeyer on the structure and innervation of the larynx. On his return to Tokyo, Taguchi became professor of the first division in the Anatomy

[27] *Brief History of Anatomy at Tokyo Imperial University, Ika Daigaku* (Tokyo Medical Society, Twenty-Five Years).

Institute, while Koganei Ryosei directed the second division. Koganei's major research interest was anthropology.

Taguchi published a series of five articles on the structure of the orbit and the relationships of the ophthalmic artery and its branches to the optic foramen. In 1893 he wrote an interesting history of anatomy, in which he emphasized its historic role as the basis for medicine.[28] Taguchi was honored by being elected president of the first Japan Medical Congress in 1902, and he continued to be an active and productive member of the faculty until his death in 1904.

Taguchi assisted Leopold Mueller and then Joseph Donitz in the development of a collection of the skeletons of a large number of animals. At his death in 1912, Joseph Donitz left his collection of 431 specimens to the institute.

Koganei Ryosei collected more than 1,200 specimens of the skeletons of various racial and ethnic groups of the fossil age. Thus, "by 1900 the institute had the finest, largest, and most diversified museums in Asia."[29]

The library developed to a comparable state of excellence, thanks to contributions from the German professors. Its prize section, the Waldeyer Library, contained 4,500 books and monographs donated by the renowned Berlin anatomist, who maintained a continuing liaison with Igakubu. The Fürbringer Library at the institute included reprints and dissertations contributed by Fürbringer.

Osawa Kenji first studied pharmacology, then trained as a physiologist under Helmholtz and Du Bois-Reymond. When he returned to Tokyo in 1874, he taught physics for students in the preparatory school and then in the special course. When the Berliner Ernest Tiegel joined the faculty in 1876 to teach physiology, Osawa became his assistant, and they initiated Japan's first teaching program in physiology.

Tiegel, a neurophysiologist, and Osawa collaborated on studies on the functions of the spinal cord of reptiles. In 1877, with Osawa as senior author, they published the first scientific paper from a Japanese laboratory to appear in a European journal.[30]

In 1878 Osawa returned to Germany to study neurophysiology with Friedrich L. Goltz (1834-1902) and medical chemistry with Felix Hoppe-Selyer (1825-1895). On his return to Tokyo in 1882, after earning a doctorate, Osawa taught both medical chemistry and physiology. Tiegel re-

---

[28] Kaibogaku no yurai oyobi sono igaku no taihan taru koto (Origins of the Study of Anatomy as the Basis of Medicine (Tokyo Iji-shinsi: Saisei-gakusha Iji-shimpo, 1893), pp. 801-5.

[29] S. Nishi and R. Ura, "The Institute of Anatomy, Imperial University of Tokyo," *Methods and Problems of Education,* 16th ser. (New York: The Rockefeller Foundation, 1930), pp. 125-30.

[30] K. Osawa and E. Tiegel, "Beobachtungen über die Funktionen des Rückenmarks der Schlangen, aus dem Physiologischen Laboratorium zu Tokyo," *Archiv für die gesamte Physiologie,* 1878, *16:* 90-100.

turned to Germany the same year, and Osawa became the first Japanese to lecture in physiology and to lead the program.

Osawa was a prolific investigator; his main studies were on the spinal reflexes and spinal nerves, as well as on the physiological bases of right- and left-handedness. His interests led him to other fields, and he wrote papers on reproduction, group movement, nutrition, and hygiene.

Osawa Kenji continued to teach medical chemistry until 1890, when Kumakawa Muneo (1839-1902) returned after five years of postgraduate study of physiological chemistry in Berlin with Ernst Salkowski. He was appointed *Koshi* (lecturer), but his first year was wasted because there was neither space nor equipment for teaching medical chemistry—and also no budget. In January 1891, an area in the physiology laboratories was turned over to Kumakawa, where he instituted a course for second-year medical students, giving lectures and demonstrations in urine analysis. In 1893, medical chemistry was established as a separate department, but it was not until 1896 that adequate financial support was made available for developing a proper program.

Anton Johannes Cornelis Geerts (1843-1883), a Hollander, is honored for his work in pharmacy and drug control, and as the author of the first Japanese pharmacopoeia.[31] Born in Oudendijk, on March 20, 1843, Geerts trained in chemistry and pharmacy and taught those subjects at the Army Medical School in Utrecht. During this period, he prepared his first publication, a textbook on qualitative and quantitative chemistry. At the suggestion of Dr. A.W.M. van Hasselt, chief of the Health Division of the Dutch Army, Geerts went to Nagasaki in the summer of 1869, where he taught chemistry and physics at Yoka, the preparatory school of the Nagasaki medical school.

His suspicions of the quality of imported medicines were first aroused in 1873, when he analyzed two imported bottles of quinine sulfate and found that they had been adulterated. A bottle supposed to contain potassium iodide instead contained brown potash, and samples of imported drugs bearing English, French, and American labels were bogus or adulterated. He found that there were no controls whatsoever over the flow of drugs into Nagasaki. Furthermore, drugs were peddled indiscriminately on the lanes and in the shops.

Geerts advised the Nagasaki government in 1873 to apply tight controls to all drugs and to establish a testing laboratory to assure their quality; this was the beginning of drug control in Japan.[32] Geerts moved to Tokyo in March 1874 and with George Martin, a German, established *Shiyakujo,* a national drug-control office sponsored by Mombusho. It was later transferred to the campus of the Tokyo Igakko. Rules for

[31] Shimizu Totaro, "Dr. A.J.C. Geerts (1843-83), a Dutch Pharmacist in Japan," *Journal of Practical Pharmacy,* September 1964, *15:* 107-11.

[32] *Nagasaki Igaku Hyakunenshi* (1961), p. 168.

controlling poisonous drugs were established, along with quality controls. Because of the frequent adulteration of quinine sulfate and potassium iodide, specific measures stated that the stocking and sale of inferior products were forbidden and that violaters would be fined. In December 1874, the hygiene office promulgated a law establishing tight controls over all drugs, and one month later, free tests for the purity of quinine sulfate and potassium iodide became available at *Shiyakujo.*

In February 1875, a second *Shiyakujo* was established in Kyoto, with Geerts as director; and the following month, a similar laboratory opened in Osaka. In all three laboratories, trained chemists were employed to test drinking water, mineral waters, and the waters of spas.

After Kyoto *Shiyakujo* was closed in August 1876, Geerts became director of Yokohama *Shiyakujo* on January 1, 1877. At both the Kyoto and the Yokohama *Shiyakujo,* Geerts taught hygiene and pharmacy to the officers of those bureaus and to the technical staff. By 1876, a comprehensive drug-control program was operating in Japan.

In 1875, at the request of the hygiene bureau (*Eisei Kyoku*), Geerts began, together with Dwars, another Hollander, to compile *Nippon Yakkyokuho* (Japanese pharmacopoeia). Geerts based the text on European sources, and it was completed in four volumes in December 1877, after Dwars had returned to the Netherlands.

Geerts was a man of multiple interests. He planned the improvement of mineral springs at Arima and Atami, and, from his studies of mineral springs across Japan, published *Nippon Kosenki* (record of Japanese mineral springs).

Geerts also wrote *Honzo Komoku* (section of minerals), two volumes in French, with Chinese characters for specific names. Volume one (published by Levy; Yokohama 1878), was dedicated to J.k.H. De Ros van Alderwelt, war minister of the Netherlands, to Okubo Toshimichi (1830-1878), and to Ichijo, a leading counselor of the Meiji government and minister of the interior. It includes sections on hydrogen, sulfur, arsenic, and carbon. The second volume (published by Levy and S. Salabelle; Yokohama, 1883) includes chapters on silicates, light metals, and heavy metals. Geerts was completing a third volume, with discussions of organic substances, fossils, and luminescent minerals, when he died suddenly on August 3, 1883.

Geerts was buried in Yamate, Yokohama, and on August 30, 1891, a monument to his memory was unveiled in Tennoji cemetery, Yanaka, Shitaya, Tokyo. It bears the following legend, endorsed by Nagayo Sensai:

Stationed in Yokohama, you took charge of infectious-disease control, at the request of the Kanagawa prefectural government. The establishment of a disinfection unit with an isolation hospital are due to your able administration. When there was a cholera epidemic in the Kansai area in 1877, you inspected all personnel entering Yokohama harbor by establishing the regulation that all ships must go through quarantine. Your work with prefectural officials resulted in excellent administration. You drafted the articles of the infectious-disease-control mission and submitted them to the minister of the interior. In recognition of your distinguished service, you were decorated with the Fourth Order of Merit of the Rising Sun. You passed away suddenly at the age of forty-three. You fostered the prospering of our medicine and assured the quality of our drugs, and yet you have left before you could see the implementation of the regulation for physicians and pharmacists, and the revision of the law on infectious-disease control. What a loss!

Education and research in pharmacology had their origins with the founding of the Institute of Pharmacology/Pharmacy in 1875. The first director, Alexander Langgard (1847-1917), studied at the pharmacological institute in Berlin and after four years accepted an invitation to come to Tokyo, where he established the first curriculum and research in pharmacy. He also gave occasional lectures to the medical students. Laggard wrote the first version of a *Pharmacopoeia Japonica;* a complete Japanese pharmacopoeia was not published until 1887, and it was based largely on Langgard's manuscript.

On his return to Berlin in 1881, Langgard was appointed to the staff of the institute in Berlin, along with Liebreich. Langgard was a prolific writer and is best-known for his pocket handbook.[33]

Instruction in pharmacology at Igakujo was offered informally in a few occasional lectures. J. J. Eijkman, a German chemist at the pharmacy institute, lectured in the early 1880s, but it was not until 1885, when Takahashi Juntaro returned from postgraduate studies in Germany, that a formal program in pharmacology could be established. Since there was no space for his program in the medical-school buildings, Takahashi used three rooms in the abandoned students' dormitory as classroom and laboratory. After one year, he was promoted to a full professorship and, with increased financial support, acquired an adequate supply of textbooks and laboratory equipment. The program moved to different laboratories on several occasions and in 1902 finally obtained its own institute.

Pathology was limited to allusions in lectures in other disciplines until Miyake Hiizu (also Shu) (1848-1938) returned from his studies in Europe in April 1877 and initiated lectures on the subject. He was the son of Miyake Gonsai, a *Rangakusha,* and had learned English from J. C. Hepburn, the distinguished American missionary-ophthalmologist, and then served as interpreter for Mueller and Hoffmann. In 1874 he completed the translation of *San-ron (Discourse in Midwifery* circa 1775) by Kagawa Genetsu, which was the major text for Japanese obstetricians who followed the practices of *Kampo.*[34] Miyake divided the translation into four sections: (1) development

---

[33] A. Langgard and O. Liebreich, *Medizinisches Rezept-Taschenbuch.* See *Biographisches Lexikon der hervorragenden Ärzte der letzten 50 Jahre,* ed. Dr. I Fischer (Berlin, 1932).

[34] The translation, with comments by Mueller, was published in "Über die japanische Gerburtshülfe," *Mitteilungen der Deutschen Gesellschaft für Natur- und Volkerkunde,* September 1874, *5:* 21-27; September 1875, *8:* 9-13; and July 1876, *10:* 9-16.

of the embryo and gestation, (2) choice of locale and position of woman during labor, (3) postpartum care, and (4) use of obstetrical chair and an abdominal binder.

A practitioner diagnosed pregnancy by placing his fingertips against those of the patient. If the pulsations in the fingertips and those in the posterior tibial artery were stronger than the pulse in the raidal artery, the patient was presumed to be pregnant. The sex of the fetus was indicated by its position in the uterus; if it was on the right side, it was a male; if on the left side, a female.

If a patient aborted within the first three months of gestation, the tissue of the embryo had five different colors, affirming the belief that the human body is the essence of the five elements of *Chung-i* (Chinese traditional medicine): water, fire, metal, wood, and earth.

Medication was based on mixtures with a number of ingredients; for example, a decoction to stimulate the flow of milk from the breast contained nine ingredients including cinnamon, euonymus, and flowers of the peony. Ancient texts decried the use of a binder as comparable to placing a heavy stone upon a young plant and stunting its growth. They also considered massage harmful and compared it with continually manipulating the roots of any young plant: invariably, growth would be retarded and the plant would die.

Miyake described the structure and use of an instrument developed by Kagawa Mitsutaka, grandson of the author of *San-ron,* known by foreigners as a "whalebone sling." In difficult labor a length of cord was passed around the fetus, and at times delivery was thereby facilitated, but since that sling frequently injured the fetus, its use was not permitted at the royal court. Therefore, Kagawa Mitsutaka developed a cloth forceps that consisted of a piece of cloth rolled on two slender rods. They were slipped into the pelvic canal and the cloth unrolled around the head of the fetus. The rods were then withdrawn, and the ends of the two pieces of cloth were threaded through a hole in a piece of whalebone, which was then used for traction. This way, the fetus was seldom injured.

Miyake Hiizu established the first series of lectures in the history of Western medicine in 1883. In the same year Imamura Ryoan began instruction in the history of Chinese and Japanese medicine.

For more than one decade the development of other academic programs had a higher priority than pathological anatomy, and as a sign of its lowly status, that subject was the last on the list of questions in the examinations. When Koganei Ryosei (or Yoshikiyo) assumed leadership in anatomy in 1885, Joseph Disse left the program to institute the first organized teaching program in pathological anatomy.

In March 1887, Miura Moriharu returned from Germany and succeeded Disse. After graduating from Igakubu, Miura had gone to Germany on his own funds, but his abilities were brought to the attention of *Mombusho,* and the ministry awarded him a scholarship. It stipulated that he would prepare himself for an academic career in pathology and pathological anatomy. He studied with Virchow in Berlin.

Yamagiwa Katsusaburo (1863-1930) became head of pathological anatomy in 1894, after three years (1891-1894) of study in Germany. He compiled a thorough description of the programs in pathology and pathological anatomy (*The History and Development of Japanese Pathology after the First Publication of the Society's Journal*).

General pathology was taught five hours a week for three semesters, followed by pathological anatomy, for which a similar block of time was assigned. Systemic pathology extended over two semesters for four hours a week. As in all the other programs, the lecture received greater emphasis than in the German schools, while the time allotted for demonstrations was sharply reduced.

Yamagiwa compared pathology curricula in Japan, Germany, and the United States, with the following results:

	Japan	Germany	United States
Lecture	213 hours	160 hours	88 hours
Practical	88 hours	50 hours	145 hours
Demonstrations	45 hours	170 hours	74 hours

The major texts were *Die Cellular-pathologie in ihrer Begrundung auf physiologische und pathologische Gewebelehre* (1858) of Rudolf Virchow and *Handbuch der pathologischen Anatomie* (1842-1846) of Karl Rokitansky. All equipment in the teaching laboratory was from Germany, including forty high-quality Zeiss microscopes. Most of the corpses for autopsies came from Ichigaya prison; there were eighty-five in 1887 and eighty-three the following year. Other autopsy material came from the teaching hospital and Yoikuin, a nearby orphanage. Research programs focused primarily on the special disease problems of Japan: schistosomiasis, *kakke,* hydatid disease, actinomycosis, and tuberculosis of the spine.

Yamagiwa accompanied Ogata Masanori on the plague expedition to Formosa in 1898. His major contribution was in carcinogenesis, for which he achieved international renown. In 1914 Yamagiwa, assisted by Ichikawa Koichi, proved that coal tar will induce a malignant tumor on the ear of a rabbit: it was the first artificially induced cancer. For this he received the highest award of the imperial academy in 1919, and in 1928, a comparable decoration from the German scientific community.

The concept of a university in which all instruction would be in Japanese was advanced by *Mombusho* in 1875-1877. The school would be located in Ichikawa Konodai in Chiba prefecture, to be Japan's own "true" university. But the plan was abandoned because of the creation of Tokyo University in 1877 and the expenses of the Seinan Wars in the same year.

In May 1877, Tokyo Igakko was merged with Kaisei Gakko to form Tokyo Daigaku (Tokyo University), with a single administrative officer. Erwin Baelz found his German colleagues suspicious of the move; they feared that by establishing the new faculties, the Japanese planned to replace the German teachers with a staff from Britain.[35]

The first graduation took place in April 1879, students were awarded *Igakushi,* and the medical school and hospital were dedicated a few weeks later, two and a half years after they had been opened. The ceremonies were made illustrious by the attendance of the emperor. Schultze and Baelz were irritated that the speeches by the Japanese included no mention of appreciation for the role of the Germans in establishing and developing the programs, but an official message from the emperor a few days later that saluted their success was balm to their psychic wounds: "His majesty, the emperor, was very pleased to observe the excellent institution and the progress of the study of medicine. There is no doubt that this success is due to the devoted work of you and the other professors. . . . The high officials who accompanied the emperor were equally astonished at the excellent state of affairs."[36]

The student attrition rate was high. For example, 129 first-year students were enrolled in 1874; by 1877 their number had dwindled to 31, and only 20 graduated in 1884.

The first foreign influences during the Meiji period, as expressed in the Education Law of 1872, which established education as compulsory, were derived from the French, who favored a standardized and centralized system. Many obstacles to educational development existed in Japan, including shortages of teachers, textbooks, and buildings.

The Iwakura mission (1871-1873) undertook a firsthand analysis of educational systems in America. Its work was continued by the first Japanese ambassador to America, Mori Arinori (1847-1889), who had been a member of the group of young men sent from Satsuma to study in Britain in 1865. He was appointed to the ambassadorial post in Washington in 1870. Soon after his arrival, Mori made a comprehensive study of the American system, and his findings, built on the observations of the Iwakura mission, placed American educators in an influential position.

Professor David Murray, Ph.D. (1830-1905), of Rutgers University, came to Tokyo in 1873 and spent six years as chief advisor to Mombusho and director of educational administration. Murray spent his first year studying the new educational system and analyzing the needs of the empire. His recommendations at the conclusion of his study were that all instruction

[35] Baelz, *Awakening Japan,* p. 33.
[36] Letter from Tanaka Fujimaro, vice-minister of education, April 30, 1879.

should be in Japanese and that normal schools should be established to train Japanese, who would replace the foreign teachers. At that time, there were fifty-one Japanese and forty-six foreign teachers.[37] Murray also recommended that Japanese textbooks should be prepared as rapidly as possible and a program developed for the education of females.

Because of the strong American influence, English became the required foreign language in the secondary schools and higher-educational institutions. Subsequently, in the 1880s, *Mombusho* required that English be taught also in the primary schools.

But by 1880, the Prussian influence began to permeate the educational system with its philosophy that the purpose of education was to train the individual to serve the state rather than to meet his own needs. Education became totally centralized, and in December of that year, a new law decreed that every aspect of education would be determined and administered by *Mombusho*. Furthermore, after 1888, any major changes had to be approved by the Privy Council, made up of the emperor's most trusted advisors. Thus, Prussian nationalism and bureaucracy became the basis of the educational system. Henceforth Tokyo University was the exclusive training ground for higher posts in the diplomatic service and in the judicial and executive branches of the government. In contrast with applicants for other positions in government and private enterprises, candidates there were not required to pass qualifying examinations.

By the University Ordinance of 1886, Tokyo attained full university status as an imperial university, Teikoku Daigaku, with faculties of medicine, engineering, law, literature, and science under a single administration. The name of the medical school was changed from Igakubu (department of medicine) to Ika Daigaku (medical college). A graduate research division corresponding to a graduate school had been created in 1880.

Tokyo University became the mecca for promising young Japanese men throughout the country. The School of Law, previously under the Ministry of Justice, and the College of Engineering, formerly under the Ministry of Public Works, were integrated as university faculties. Only three of the national institutions of higher and specialized education remained independent: Sapporo Agricultural School, Tokyo Forestry School, and Komaba Agricultural School. By the 1890s, however, the latter two institutions were merged into Tokyo University, and by 1885, the university had expanded into a comprehensive institution consisting of five faculties: law and politics, literature, science, engineering, and medicine, with a total enrollment of over 1,000 students. As Japanese students returned from abroad and became teachers at Tokyo University, the ideal of the "true" Japanese university came to full fruition at the beginning of the twentieth century.

[37] Hugh Borton, *Japan's Modern Century*, 2nd ed. (New York: The Ronald Press, 1970), p. 203.

As a result of the expansion of secondary education came increased demands for higher education, which only Tokyo University could meet. Moreover, education recognized a growing demand by industries for qualified graduates from institutions of higher learning. The government, therefore, decided as early as 1894 to revise school regulations in order to convert the higher schools, formerly used for preparing students for the university, into institutions offering specialized education. But this measure did not survive, and by 1901, the higher schools were once again preparing students for the university.

For a long time, Tokyo University remained the sole university and was regarded as the only institution for higher education and for academic research. The Diet passed measures to meet the growing demand for higher education, and a second imperial university was established in Kyoto in 1897. In the following twenty years, imperial universities were established at Sendai, Fukuoka, and Sapporo.

When Wilhelm Schultze returned to Prussia, he was succeeded by Julius Karl Scriba (1848-1905), who became a close friend of Erwin Baelz and shared his affection for Japan and the Japanese. Scriba was born June 5, 1848, at Weinheim, Hesse. After attending a *Gymnasium* at Darmstadt, he enrolled in the faculty of medicine at Heidelberg. His studies were interrupted by the Franco-Prussian War, at the end of which he was decorated by his *Land* for bravery. Scriba completed postgraduate studies in abdominal surgery at Heidelberg with Vincenz Czerny (1842-1916), a leading protégé of Billroth. He then studied at the surgical/gynecological clinic of Gustav Siemans (1824-1876) at Freiburg. Siemans was the first to attempt total nephrectomy, an operation that Scriba introduced to Japan in 1888. Scriba completed his *Habilitationsschrift*, "Investigation of Fat Embolism," at Leipzig in 1879 and two years later, on June 5, 1881, arrived at Tokyo. Sato Susumu, Hashimoto Tsunatsune, and Takagi Kanehiro, all of whom had studied in Germany, became his principal associates.

Scriba enjoyed teaching, and the students preferred his clear, precise, and measured presentations to the hurried style of Erwin Baelz, which made note taking difficult. Since full-time teaching posts in a number of specialties were still unfilled, Scriba taught medical jurisprudence, dermatology, syphilology, and ophthalmology, as well as general surgery.

According to the testimony of his devoted associate, Dohi Keizo, he was thoughtful and selfless in his relations with his students and his staff. A genial man, Scriba enjoyed entertaining his colleagues. He was an unusually dexterous surgeon. Dohi described his nimble fingers as "dancing," and added that Scriba had the mind of a Buddha and the hands of a priest.[38] Scriba developed a large and affluent practice; he saw private patients at his home three afternoons a week. Furthermore, he broke the long-standing tradition of charging no fees by billing for his services and asking patients

[38] Dohi Keizo, *Gakken Yugi* (Tokyo: Kaizosha, 1927), p. 380.

to pay him directly. As his surgical renown spread, patients were referred to him from Shanghai, Manila, Hong Kong, Singapore, and Vladivostok.

Botany held a special attraction for Scriba, and while he was still a student in Heidelberg, he published an essay on the flowers and plants of Hesse, "Flora der Bluten und höheren Sproen-Pflanzen des Grossherzogtum Hesse unter der angrenzenden Gebiete" (Darmstadt, 1873). He published a second article on the same subject five years later. In Tokyo, he developed an extensive botanical collection from Sakhalin, Taiwan, China, and Korea, as well as Japan. Scriba was coauthor of *Enumeratio Plantarum,* listing 2,743 species of 1,035 genera of Japanese plants.

One of Scriba's most valuable collections was fifty-five antique Japanese gold and silver coins. In a lecture in 1888 to the Deutsche Gesellschaft entitled "Bemerkungen über japanische Gold- und Silbermünzen," he traced the history of various coins dating back to 1600. Scriba illustrated his lecture with charts of the dates of the usage of the coins on both the Japanese and Christian calendars, their name and weight, the content of precious metals and alloys, and the estimated value in Mexican dollars.

Scriba played a major role in the development of excellent military medicine and surgery. The results first became evident to the world during the Russo-Japanese War (February 8 to September 5, 1905).

The first scientific meeting of the professors and assistant professors was held in September 1884. It consisted of concise reports on research programs and discussions. Henceforth the meetings were held weekly from six until nine in the evening.

The following year, the medical students formed Toyo Igakukai (or Igakkai) (Oriental medical society) with the aim of advancing medicine in the Far East. The monthly meetings were both academic and social, with membership open to all students.

In September 1885, the first discussions were held on the possibility of merging the two societies, but this was not accomplished until 1887. The first meeting of the merged societies, now known as Tokyo Igakukai (or Igakkai), was held in January 1888. The chairman and counselors were from the faculty, and a handful of students were appointed assistants. Miyake Hiizu, a pathologist, served the first two-year term as chairman, 1888-1890, and Osawa Kenji, as the first editor of the society's proceedings. Osawa succeeded Miyake as chairman from 1890 to 1894, and he, in turn, was succeeded by Koganei Ryosei (or Yoshikiyo).

When Erwin Baelz departed on home leave in December 1884, W. van der Heyeden (d. 1894) served as his replacement. After completing medical studies at Utrecht, Van der Heyeden taught and practiced medicine in Kobe and in Niigata, on the Japan Sea. He returned to the Netherlands for postgraduate studies and then practiced in Yokohama, where he carried out morphological studies of the formed elements of the blood of Japanese.

During his year at Igakubu, Van der Heyeden worked with Julius Scriba in establishing Nippon Yakkyoku, an institute for the advancement of pharmacy. When Baelz returned to Tokyo at the end of 1885, Van der Heyeden resumed his practice and studies at Yokohama until he left for Europe with a terminal illness in 1894.

Communicable diseases were the major health problems in Japan during the Meiji era. There were severe epidemics of cholera in 1877-1879, 1881-82, 1885-86, and 1898, owing to cases entering at Nagasaki and Yokohama from China. Cholera was widespread in Kyushu in 1879 and extended as far north as Tokyo; of an estimated 160,000 cases, there were 100,000 fatalities. An equally high mortality rate was associated with the epidemic in 1886: 155,155 cases, with 109,758 deaths.

In the early years of the Meiji era, dysentery was confined to Kyushu and Shikoku, but in 1893 it spread to Tokyo, with 160,000 cases that year. There were recurrent outbreaks of typhus fever in 1880, 1885, 1886, and 1887, with 8,225 cases and 1,577 deaths recorded in 1886.

Although vaccination against smallpox was made compulsory in 1876, implementation of the regulation was slow. There were 73,337 cases in 1886, with 18,678 deaths, and 12,176 deaths in an epidemic of 41,946 cases in 1897.

The government and educated citizens were haunted by the spectre of continuing epidemics. Fortunately, several of Japan's finest scientific minds established careers in bacteriology and contributed important new knowledge on several bacterial diseases. Research and training in bacteriology developed along two pathways: at Densembyo Kenkyujo (Institute for Infectious Diseases), and at the Bacteriology and Hygiene Institute of the medical school.

Before the flowering of bacteriology under Louis Pasteur and Robert Koch in the last quarter of the nineteenth century, education and research in hygiene were linked to physiology. So it was that the first lectures in hygiene were given by Ernest Tiegel, a physiologist who had a special interest in the field. After Tiegel's departure in 1882, Katayama Kuniyoshi, assistant professor of forensic medicine, lectured on hygiene until 1884, when Osawa Kenji took over for one year. Erwin Baelz also emphasized the importance of hygienic practices in his lectures in internal medicine and obstetrics.

Hygiene was merged with the new field of bacteriology with the return from Germany of Ogata Masanori (1852-1919), who joined the faculty in January 1885. Ogata had first studied medicine at Jishukan, a school for traditional medicine in Kumamoto, also known as Higo (fief), in west central Kyushu. It had opened in 1756 as Saishunkan under the sponsorship of the *daimyo*, Hosokawa Shigekata, and was one of the earliest medical schools sponsored by a *han* for the teaching of *Kampo*. Jishukan was closed with the Meiji restoration, and the *daimyo,* Hosokawa Morihisa, sponsored the establishment of Igakusho, a school to teach Western medicine at which, as we have seen, C. J. Mansvelt taught from 1870 to 1874. Kitasato Shibasaburo (1856-1931), Japan's greatest bacteriologist, was a fellow student of Ogata at Kumamoto, and their careers were intertwined in both friendship and disagreement.

Ogata moved to Tokyo in 1871 and enrolled at Igakubu, where he graduated in 1881. The following year, 1882-3, as a *ryugakusei* ("foreign-study student"), he studied at the imperial health office's Physiological Institute in Berlin. This was just two years after the arrival of Robert Koch, who had been serving as district physician at Wallstein in East Prussia. At Wallstein, Koch conducted his epochal studies on spore formation by anthrax bacilli, which drew wide acclaim when he reported them at Breslau in April 1876. In Berlin, Ogata learned the fundamentals of bacteriology and basic laboratory techniques.

After one year, Ogata moved to the Institute of Hygiene in Munich, headed by Max von Pettenkoffer (1818-1901). Founded in 1866, Pettenkoffer's institute was the first center where laboratory methods were rigorously applied in the investigation of hygiene and public health. He was also the first to develop studies on the hygienic aspects of nutrition: water, sewage, ventilation, and clothing. Here Ogata developed techniques for the pure culture of pathogenic and nonpathogenic bacteria. His contributions were heralded by Pettenkoffer in 1897, when Ogata visited Munich after the World Medical Congress in Moscow.

At a reception in Ogata's honor, Pettenkoffer told the guests that Ogata was the pioneer of bacteriology at the hygiene institute in Munich.[39] Pettenkoffer had been the last important exponent of the miasmatic theory of epidemics, and Ogata's studies were an early stimulus for Pettenkoffer to turn to the application of laboratory methods in public health and hygiene.

Governmental supervision of public health was instituted under the direction of Sagara Chian in the medical section of the government education office, *Daigaku.* In 1872 *Daigaku* became *Mombusho* (education ministry), and three years later the administration of public health was transferred to the section of police administration in *Naimusho* (home ministry). Nagayo Sensai succeeded Sagara and was director of the Public Health Office until 1891. Unfortunately, medical education and research were permanently separated from public health.[40]

After Ogata Masanori joined the medical faculty in 1885, he also conducted research at Eisei.

Shikenjo (the Tokyo Hygiene Laboratory) was under the directorship of Nagayo Sensai and *Naimusho.* Kitasato Shibasaburo, who was one of Ogata's five assistants in the laboratory, was born on December 20, 1852,

[39] *Tokyo Medical Society, Twentyfive Years,* p. 116.
[40] Responsibility for public health today rests in *Kaiseijo* (health ministry).

the son of a *samurai* of the Kumamoto fief. After studying at Igakujo from 1871 to 1874, Kitasato enrolled at Tokyo Igakko, where he graduated in 1883. He then worked as assistant to Nagayo Sensai in the Public Health office, and when Ogata joined the research laboratory in January 1885, at his request Kitasato became his assistant. Together they studied the possibility of a bacterial etiology for *kakke*. The same year, Kitasato went to Koch's laboratory in Berlin under the sponsorship of the Public Health office, where he gained international renown before his return to Tokyo in 1892.

Although they were boyhood friends in Kumamoto and worked together in Tokyo, Ogata and Kitasato became engaged in a series of scientific disputes, which contributed to the intense rivalry that developed between the medical faculty and Kitasato. The animosity began when Ogata published his report that he had isolated a specific microorganism as the etiological agent of *kakke*.[41] Ogata's reports were evaluated by Robert Koch and his deputy, Frederick A. J. Loeffler (1852-1915).[42]

Koch and Loeffler concluded that Ogata's claims were false and because he was Japanese asked Kitasato to publish a rebuttal in Japanese and German. This placed Kitasato on the horns of a dilemma, because he had studied under Ogata in the public-health research laboratory, and a strong Japanese tradition forbade one to criticize one's teachers. When Kitasato pointed out his problem to Koch, the latter insisted that as a true scientist, Kitasato should never allow his personal relationships to interfere with the forward march of science. Although Kitasato's refutation of Ogata's claims was carefully couched in terms that avoided personal criticism, it was seized on by the conservative members of the medical faculty at Igakubu as a flagrant violation of the cardinal principles of conduct.

Kitasato and Robert Koch shared a passion for hard work, and Kitasato became closer to Koch than any of his German students did. Kitasato's devotion to the research bench led to a remarkable record of scientific achievements during his years with Koch. In 1889 he obtained the first pure culture of tetanus bacilli, and the following year, Kitasato and Von Behring proved that injections of diphtheria toxin protected against the disease. This initiated the treatment of infectious diseases with serum therapy based on the production of antitoxins by toxins.

In 1891 Von Behring and Kitasato reported in *Deutsche medizinische Wochenschrift* the development of immunity to tetanus based on the injection of mice and rabbits with tetanus cultures.

When Kitasato attended the London Hygiene Congress of 1891, he shared star billing with Joseph Lister, Pierre Paul Émile Roux (1853-1933) of the Pasteur Institute, who shared the Nobel Prize with Von Behring for

[41] Ogata Masanori, "Untersuchungen über die Etiologie der *Kak'ke*," *Ärztliches Intelligenzblatt*, 1885, *32*: 683-86.

[42] Loeffler and Edwin Krebs (1834-1913) were codiscovers of *Cornybacterium diphtheriae* in 1884.

his research on diphtheria toxin, and Elie Metchnikoff (1845-1916), who made the first transmission of syphilis to an experimental animal and was also a pioneer contributor to cellular immunity.

After the congress, Kitasato was offered an appointment as director of the bacteriological section of the pathological institute in Cambridge. He declined on the grounds that he felt an obligation to return to Japan because of the support he had received from the government. By now he had become to the first foreigner to be appointed to a professorship at Berlin University.

Kitasato returned to Tokyo in early 1892 and rejoined the Public Health Office under Nagayo Sensai, but he soon became dissatisfied and sought his own bacteriological-research institute. Nagayo Sensai presented the issue to Fukuzawa Yukichi, who, in his advocacy of Western studies, had told friends that he would assist a few scientists to establish permanent careers. Fukuzawa gave a plot of land in Tokyo and 2,000 Yen for equipment. but when *Mombusho* presented a request to the Diet for the new facility, Densembyo Kenkyujo (Institute for Infectious Diseases), to be erected at Tokyo University next to Ogata Masanori's institute, it encountered violent opposition sparked by leaders of Tokyo University. Kitasato desired an institute without governmental controls, and it began as a program of the Great Japan Hygiene Society, of which Hasegawa, vice-director of the medical school, 1872-1874, was a director. As a member of the Diet and a strong backer of Kitasato, Hasegawa had become influential, and Kitasato also generated considerable public support because of the anxieties over the continuing problem of communicable diseases in Japan.

Another dimension was added to the conflict between the medical faculty and Kitasato by the antagonism that his insistence on an autonomous institute now generated in *Mombusho*. On Kitasato's return from Berlin, Nagayo Sensai and Ishiguro Tadanori, president of the Central Hygiene Commission, proposed that the chair of hygiene and bacteriology be divided to create a professorship for Kitasato as well as for Ogata. Such an arrangement existed in several other disciplines, but *Mombusho* refused to approve such an arrangement for Kitasato. Kitasato's insistence on autonomy thwarted two other efforts by the medical faculty to bring him into the fold. When their plans for an institute of infectious diseases were being implemented in November 1892, Osawa Kenji, as the *Bucho* (dean), offered the directorship to Kitasato, but his terms were unacceptable to the faculty. Five years later Dean Aoyama Tanemichi initiated a second offer to Kitasato, but *Mombusho* refused to approve it.

For Kitasato, the most damaging dispute with the medical faculty concerned his claim to the first identification of the plague bacillus. Conventional wisdom has it that Kitasato and Alexandre Jean-Emil Yersin

(1863-1943) independently and almost simultaneously discovered the plague bacillus, *Pasteurella pestis*, during an epidemic in Hong Kong in 1894.

Yersin, a French-speaking Swiss, was born in Rougemont, Canton Vaud, near Lausanne, on September 22, 1863. He studied medicine in Lausanne and Marburg. His thesis, "Study on the Development of Experimental Tuberculosis," opened his career in bacteriology. In the same year he joined the Pasteur Institute, where he made a deep impression: "Pasteur had long recognized the very great qualities in the pupil, whose habits of labor were almost those of an ascete."[43] Yersin assisted Pierre P. E. Roux (1853-1933) in his studies in 1888, which showed that bacteria-free filtrates from broth cultures of the diphtheria bacillus produced lesions characteristic of diphtheria and death in animals rendered susceptible to the bacillus. This led to serotherapy based on the conclusion that the bacillus produces its effects through an exotoxin and that the disease can be treated effectively with an antitoxin.

Yersin then became a naval surgeon in the French colonial forces and director of the Pasteur Institute at Nha-Trand, Amman, and later at Saigon, French Indochina. He came to Hong Kong in 1894 to study the plague and to find the most effective means of preventing its spread to the French colonies. Yersin observed that most cases were among Chinese who lived in rat-infested slums, and he inoculated rats, mice, and guinea pigs with blood and pulp from infected lymph nodes of human victims. He isolated the causative bacillus from the spleen and blood of infected animals and concluded that plague was a contagious disease transmissible by inoculation. Although he had determined that rats were the principal vehicle, Yersin recognized that fleas could also transmit the disease.

After he returned to Paris in 1895, Yersin developed a plague serum, which he employed with some success in Indochina the following year.[44] The decision of the Japanese government to send a team to investigate the etiology of the disease in Hong Kong started a bitter controversy over its membership. A bacteriologist and a clinician would be appropriate members of such a study group. In a move that was largely self-serving, the chauvinistic wing of the medical faculty argued for the designation of Ogata Masanori and Aoyama Tanemichi of the Institute of Internal Medicine. But the director of the school, Koganei Ryosei (or Yoshikiyo), placed scientific prowess above chauvinism and selected Kitasato to lead a team with Aoyama and Ishigami Toru from the Institute of Infectious Diseases.

Kitasato carried his obsession with autonomy to Hong Kong, and when Yersin requested permission to autopsy corpses of plague victims in

[43] R. Vallery-Radot. *The Life of Pasteur*, trans. R. L. Devonshire (New York: Doubleday, Page & Co., 1927), p. 457.

[44] A. Yersin, "La peste boubonique à Hong Kong avec la planche XII," *Annales de L'Institut Pasteur, Journal de Microbiologie*, 1894, *8:* 662-67.

Kitasato's laboratory, he was summarily rejected. In 1894, Kitasato cabled Tokyo that he had identified the causative agent of plague and sent a preliminary communication to *The Lancet*.[45] At about the same time, Yersin identified a microorganism with quite different characteristics from Kitasato's bacillus. Kitasato's bacillus was gram-positive, motile, resembled a diplococcus, and coagulated with milk and agar. The medical faculty, led by Ogata Masanori, rejected Kitasato's claim of priority on the grounds that his bacillus did not invade the bloodstream and was gram-positive. This suggests that his cultures were probably contaminated.

Ogata became more deeply involved in 1896 when he and Yamagiwa Katsusaburo (1863-1930) of the Pathology Institute investigated an outbreak of plague in Taiwan, which had been ceded to Japan by China in the Treaty of Shimonoseki, April 17, 1895, to terminate the Sino-Japanese War.

Yamagiwa graduated from Igakubu in 1889 and spent three years, 1891 to 1894, in postgraduate studies in pathology in Germany. When he returned to Tokyo in November 1895, he was awarded the *Igaku Hakase* and was appointed professor of general pathology and pathological anatomy. His main research interest was in paragonomiasis, the lung-fluke disease.

Ogata reported that he had isolated a bacillus from patients, rats, and fleas that was identical to Yersin's bacillus; this, of course, contradicted Kitasato's claim. Yet Kitasato and Yersin continue to be credited by most authorities as the codiscoverers of the plague bacillus.[46]

In a lecture at the Deutsche Gesellschaft on December 27, 1899, Aoyama summarized much of the existing information on the plague, basing his talk on information from epidemics in Hong Kong and Bombay. After discussing the history of plague epidemics going back to the Middle East before the birth of Jesus Christ, he turned to the etiological agent and attributed its discovery to Yersin: "The disease agent of the plague was discovered during the Hong Kong epidemic by the renowned French physician Dr. Yersin. In regard to the bacillus that Dr. Kitasato discovered, as he recently admitted himself, it was not the true agent of the disease. Herewith, the honor of having discovered the plague bacillus belongs solely to Dr. Yersin."[47]

In discussing the transmission of plague, Aoyama referred to Ogata Masanori's assertion that fleas could transmit plague to humans by their bite. Ogata's statement had been the subject of continuing debate. Aoyama commented on the possibility of human infection through scratching the bite of the flea, which is today accepted as a mode of transmission.

[45] *The Lancet*, 1894, *2*: 428-30.

[46] Norman Howard-Jones in a recent article concludes that Yersin was the sole discoverer of the bacillus and that Kitasato's claims were inaccurate. He presents an interesting account of the disagreement: "Was Shibasaburo Kitasato the Codiscoverer of the Plague Bacillus?" *Perspectives in Biology and Medicine*, Winter 1973, *16*(2): 292-307.

[47] Aoyama, T., "Die Pest," *Mitteilungen der Deutschen Gesellschaft für Natur- und Volkerkunde*, 1900, *8*: 211-20.

The antagonism between Kitasato and the faculty increased as his institute rose in prestige. In 1895, it became an official agency of the Bureau of Public Health in Naimusho. There were usually eight senior scientists drawn from Todai. In 1899, the institute was given responsibility for the inspection and distribution of potentially hazardous pharmaceutical compounds, and in 1905, a monopoly over the production of smallpox vaccine. It soon became the dominant bacteriological center in the Far East.

One of the most important contributions to the conquest of disease was based upon a collaborative effort between Paul Ehrlich and Hata Sahachiro (1873-1938), a graduate of Igakubu. Hata had been associated with Kitasato and may have gone to Ehrlich's laboratory as the intermediary for the exchange of scientific information. In Frankfurt, Hata developed a system for the artificial transmission of *Treponema pallidum* to rabbits by intratesticular inoculation. Under Ehrlich's guidance, he tested chemical compounds on the mouse trypanosomiasis system and found compound number 606 (Salvarsan) to be highly effective.[48] Therefore, the compound was tested on syphilis in rabbits and it cleared their testicles of spirochetes. The first human trial was made by Hata in 1909, and the results from a single intravenous injection were dramatic. Ehrlich first announced this signal success at a scientific congress in Wiesbaden on April 19, 1910.[49]

The first specific etiological agent for bacterial dysentery was identified by Shiga Kiyoshi (1870-1957) at Kitasato's institute in 1897.[50] The son of a Sendai clan samurai, Sato Shin was adopted at the age of fifteen by Shiga Tasuke. When he had completed the study of medicine at Igakubu, Shiga joined the staff of Kitasato's institute and also served as public-health officer in the Quarantine Bureau. During an epidemic of dysentery in 1897, he identified a gram-negative bacillus in the fecal discharge of a patient with acute diarrhea. It agglutinated in the serum of patients with dysentery. However, he reported erroneously that the bacillus was motile, and it was not until three years later that Walther Kruse (1864-1943), in Germany, verified that the bacillus was nonmotile. His studies were conducted on patients with dysentery during an outbreak in the Rhine-Westphalia region. Since Kruse's bacillus was agglutinated by the same serum as Shiga's, the bacillus soon became known in some circles as the Shiga-Kruse bacillus.[51]

---

[48]P. Ehrlich and K. Shiga, "Farbentherapeutische Versuche dei Trypanosomenerkrankung," *Berliner klinische Wochenschrift,* 1904, *41* (2): 329-32; *41* (4): 362-65.

[49]P. Ehrlich and S. Hata, *Die experimentelle Chemotherapie der Spirillosen* (Berlin: Springer Verlag, 1910). An English translation was published in London in 1911. See Patrick Collard, *The Development of Microbiology* (London, New York, Melbourne: Cambridge University Press, 1976).

[50]Simon Flexner, Richard P. Strong, and W. E. Musgrave added new varieties of dysentery bacilli during an epidemic in Manila in 1900. Today this family is known as *Shigella.*

[51]"Über den Dysenteriebacillus," *Zeitschrift für Bakteriologie,* 1898, *23* (14): 599.

In May 1901, Shiga moved to Paul Ehrlich's Institut für Serumforschung in Frankfurt. He joined Ehrlich's investigations of chemotherapeutic agents in trypanosomiasis and developed a compound, trypanorol, with limited effectiveness. From Frankfurt, Shiga moved to Heidelberg, where he spent one year with Walther Albrecht Kossel (1853-1927), who was conducting pioneer studies on nucleic acids and proteins, for which he was awarded the Nobel Prize in 1910.

Shiga returned to Tokyo in 1903 and was awarded the *Igaku Hakase* in July 1905. In 1909, he conducted bacteriological studies in India under the auspices of the Japanese government, and in 1912 led a mission to Italy and England. In 1911, Shiga made a major contribution to our knowledge of beri-beri. He reported a beri-beri-like condition in various animal species, "leaving little doubt that *all* animal species are subject to the same disease when confined to dietaries of a similarly restricted type."[52]

Shiga returned to Densenbyo Kenkyusho in 1918 for one year and in April 1920 was elected professor of bacteriology at Keio University Faculty of Medicine. He was also appointed a member of the Central Health Bureau of the Ministry of the Interior. In October of that year, he was designated *Bucho* (dean) of the Keio faculty. Subsequently, he moved to Seoul as director of the Government General Hospital of Korea. On the scientific side, his principal work continued to be on serum therapy for dysentery. When Shiga retired he returned to Sendai, where he enjoyed calligraphy and writing poetry until his death in 1957 at the age of eighty-seven.

Like many Germans, Baelz took a scholarly interest in spas (*Bäder*). The Japanese were singularly devoted to bathing in steaming hot water (*O-furo*) in their homes, in public bath houses, and at spas. For them, a bath was a form of pleasure and a ritual; it was also a practical defense against the unheated Japanese buildings. Both sexes mingled naked and unashamed at home and in the public baths; age took precedence, and males bathed before females. The bather scrubbed his body and removed all suds before entering the *O-furo*.

Baelz was fascinated by *Thermalbäder* (hot springs) in Japan, of which there were some 1,000, many in remote mountain retreats.[53] At these resorts the Japanese preferred mild salty water at a temperature of 42-48° C. They usually bathed four to five times daily, but a few enjoyed as many as ten to fifteen baths a day. Patients with a tendency to internal hemorrhages and to nervous disorders were advised not to use *Thermalbäder;* for all others the baths had an intensely stimulating effect, to which Baelz applied the term *polykrato* (many effects).

[52]R. Williams, *Toward the Conquest of Beriberi* (Cambridge: Harvard University Press, 1961); quoted in Bartholomew, *The Acculturation of Science in Japan*, p. 170.

[53]E. Baelz, "Über permanente Thermalbäder," *Berliner klinischer Wochenschrift*, 1884, *21* (48): 2-3.

At Kawanaka, deep in the mountains, Baelz found a bath that he described in detail. The water was 36.2° Celsius, tasteless, and very clear. During immersion, the human body became blue-white or snow white. A few patients remained in the bath for days and even as long as weeks, around the clock, leaving the water only to perform bodily functions or to stretch. They rested in a half-lying position, or in any other comfortable position in the modest-sized wooden tubs. If a patient wished to doze, he placed a stone on his lap, so that he would not float to the surface when he fell asleep.

The caretaker at Kawanaka was a remarkable seventy-year-old man who spent practically the entire winter in the water. Although air temperatures were at the freezing mark for four to five months, he was quite comfortable in the bath with neither clothes nor a stove to warm him.

During such long periods of immersion, the skin on the hands and feet wrinkled and turned pale, like the skin of a washerwoman. The bodily functions and appetite remained normal, as did pulse and body temperature, and Baelz noticed no unpleasant subjective effects. He wished to conduct detailed metabolic studies on the long-term bathers, but because of the pressure of his tasks in Tokyo, he was unable to do so. It became clear to Baelz that such prolonged bathing did not have strong effects. He himself spent two hours uninterrupted in the bath at Kawanaka and reported that he was neither stimulated nor weakened. From this experience and his other observations he concluded that European thermal baths should be used for more extended periods. He went on to list Wildbad, Teplitz, Ragatz, and Pfäffers as *Bäder* in Germany that, because of their similarity to Kawanaka, would be quite suitable for such extended baths. They too were blessed with abundant supplies of hot water that flowed from the earth in both winter and summer. The water temperature was constant at one to two degrees below body temperature. Baelz lamented that such ideal *Bäder* went unused for the greater part of the year. Even invalids could reach them easily because good transportation was available.

Baelz saw a galaxy of therapeutic uses for these *Dauerbäder* (extended baths) in such disorders as rheumatism and other locomotor diseases; indolent burns, wounds, and abscesses; and chronic eczema and pemphigus. He recommended that the time spent in the water should vary as much as from several hours a day to weeks: "I expect tremendous success from the combination of massage and *Dauerbad* for disorders of the joints, and *Dauerbad* and localized treatment with lotions and ointments for various skin disorders."[54] He predicted that chronic pelvic discharges would also benefit from the *Dauerbad* but that only experience would reveal whether paralysis and other nervous disorders would respond favorably. Patients with actively festering wounds or similar ailments should, he thought, be segregated in a special pool.

[54] Ibid., p. 3.

While the Japanese enjoyed communal bathing, Baelz believed that Germans might find such nudity and common exposure repugnant. But he pointed out that since the water circulated constantly, inflammatory material could not pass from one person to another. Furthermore, "the idea of having company during such long baths is from the psychological standpoint decidedly preferable to solitary confinement in a water cell. The bather would not have to sit *venia verbis,* but could have the pleasure of conversation."[55]

The attraction of *Dauerbäder* would be enhanced by requiring bathers to cleanse themselves carefully before entry. He foresaw patients in Germany becoming addicted to *Dauerbäder* that had been furnished with all possible conveniences. He summarized his enthusiasm: "The *Dauerbad* is not dangerous and deserves serious trial in Germany."[56]

Baelz's investigation of *Thermalbäder* led him to Kusatsu, a tidy little town surrounded by pine and larch forests at the foot of the Shirane mountain range between Tokyo and Niigata, thirty-four miles from Karuizawa. It had been made famous as early as the twelfth century by Minamoto Yoritomo, founder of the Kamakura shogunate.[57] Kusatsu was a hot sulfur spring, or *Yunohana* ("flowers of the hot spring"), and the water also contained iron, alum, and arsenic. It was intensely hot, with a temperature as high as 147.9° F., so that the village square, where the chief public bath was located, was filled with steam. The use of the *Netsu-no-yu* (heat bath) was directed with military discipline by a bath master. The bathers reduced the temperature of the water by stirring it with long boards while they chanted a chorus. At a given signal, up to 200 bathers entered the water and remained completely motionless for three to four minutes, since physical movement would accelerate fatigue from the heat. At frequent intervals the bath master announced the amount of time remaining, and all bathers answered in a chorus.

Baelz was convinced that Kusatsu had the best mountain air in Japan and also ideal drinking water; he commented in 1904 that if he were not returning to Germany the following year, he would build a sanitorium that would attract people from all parts of the world once the unique properties of the spa became known. Patients could bathe five times daily for at least a month. Unfortunately, this would produce changes in the skin: "After about two weeks, most bathers get a purulent rash on places where the skin is soft. With continued bathing the rash improves and, if the patients spend three or four days bathing in the alkaline springs of Sawatari on the way home, the pain and severe itching decrease, and in a short time the rash

[55] Ibid.
[56] Ibid.
[57] He ruled from 1192 to 1199 and was the first in a long line of military dictators to adopt the title *Sei-i-Taishogun,* "barbarian-killing general."

heals completely."[58] Baelz was so devoted to the baths at Kusatsu that he purchased 5,700 *tsubo* of land that included a number of mineral springs.[59]

The recovery of a seriously ill patient was celebrated by the ceremony of *tokoage,* literally, "bed (or mattress) lift up." Its name was derived from the taking up from the floor of the *futon* (mattresses) upon which the patient had lain. Erwin Baelz was invited to a *tokoage* for the princess dowager of Mori, the former *daimyo* family of Choshu *han.* She had suffered an attack of apoplexy for which her Japanese physicians gave a gloomy prognosis. Baelz, however, predicted correctly that she would recover, and the family were deeply indebted to him. The leading governmental figures from Choshu, including Marquis Ito Hirobumi and Count Inouye Kaoru, also attended the *tokoage.*

The prince of Choshu occupied the seat of honor before the *tokonoma* (recessed alcove), flanked by his mother, the dowager princess, his wife, and the leading ladies of the retinue. The guests sat facing the prince and his party. They were entertained by storytellers and singers; Baelz expressed his dismay at finding *geisha* participating rather raucously in the entertainment. But the Choshu leaders told him that in their feudatory, it was quite acceptable to have *geisha* present at such a celebration. When he returned to the Kaga *yashiki,* Baelz reported in his diary that the *tokoage* was one of the most pleasant evenings that he had spent in Japan.[60]

After almost twenty years in Japan, Baelz had learned a great deal about Japanese family life. He published a revealing portrait in 1893.[61] He began by pointing out that an understanding of the Japanese life-style was made difficult by the fact that the family lived in isolation and the home was inaccessible even to close friends. He recalled the Mongoloid-Malayan origins of the Japanese and noted that two centuries earlier, Engelbert Kaempfer had traced them to the lost tribes of Israel, a derivation he inferred from the finely curved noses of the Japanese aristocrats.

In contrasting the Japanese national character with the Chinese, Baelz described the Japanese as more obliging to foreigners, but at the same time quite discreet. They differed remarkably in character from the Chinese, whom he described as "serious, reserved, opposed to all things foreign, externally conservative, very industrious, frugal to the point of greediness, very peace loving, unwarlike, and even cowardly. The Japanese is amiable,

[58] Quoted in Gerhard Vescovi, *Erwin Baelz: Wegbereiter der japanischen Medizin* (Stuttgart: A. W. Gentner Verlag, 1972), p. 64. Largely through Baelz's promotion of its virtues, Kusatsu became a well-known spa, and the citizens erected a monument to Baelz in 1935. A sister-city relationship with Bietigheim was established in 1961, and a reproduction of the Kusatsu monument to Baelz was unveiled there as a gift of Kusatsu in 1962.

[59] One *tsubo* equals six square feet.

[60] Baelz, *Awakening Japan,* pp. 126-28.

[61] E. Baelz, "Über japanisches Familienleben," *Chronik aus Schwäbischer Merkur* (19 and 22 July 1893).

courteous, cheerful, good-natured, easily delighted by new things, carefree, extravagant, frivolous, happy-go-lucky, even taking death lightly, fatalistic with a valiant disposition, courageous, and brave."[62] Baelz found these qualities to be a mixture of attractive and unattractive traits, which, added together, made a Japanese an amiable member of society.

Because of their exaggerated sense of courtesy, the Japanese tended to tell falsehoods, and truth suffered. But Baelz defended this habit as being restricted primarily to those Japanese who were foreign traders, and he suggested that the Europeans with whom they dealt exhibited the same trait but for different reasons. Furthermore, the older generation of Japanese who had grown up before extensive European contacts were true gentlemen and in no sense deceitful.

Baelz emphasized the industriousness and intellectual capacity of the Japanese; young men from prestigious families would accept employment as servants with European families in order to broaden their knowledge. The opinion of many foreign travelers that all Japanese women were of low morals was nonsense, he wrote, and was usually based on visits to the brothel areas of the port cities. Baelz compared this opinion with the reaction of a tourist to the famed houses of ill repute in Hamburg and other European seaports. One should not generalize from such sordid locales about the women of a country, he warned.

To corroborate his enthusiasm for the Japanese people, Baelz referred to the lyrical reports of Sir Edwin Arnold (1832-1904). As a staff member of the London *Daily Telegraph,* Arnold had described Japanese women as "sweet, graceful, noble, friendly, charming, quiet, and selfless," and the Japanese people as "rather of birds and butterflies than ordinary human beings."[63]

As the emperor's most trusted physician, Baelz was called repeatedly to attend the crown prince, Yoshihito, a sickly youth, and an enduring friendship between them ensued. Baelz suspected that the crown prince had a tuberculous infection of the bronchial lymph nodes, resulting from a serious bout of pneumonia in August 1895.

An interesting aspect of their warm personal relationship concerned the vital decision about the crown prince's marriage. By Japanese tradition, which Baelz decried, the emperor and the heir apparent were treated with all possible ceremony and reverence but actually had no independence whatsoever. Thus, the decision on a suitable mate for the marriage of the heir to the throne and even the date of the betrothal rested with senior statesmen. Baelz was summoned to a conference dealing with this question at the palace of Prince Takehito Arisugawa on February 8, 1900. Hashimoto Tsunatsune and Oka Genkyo, as court physicians, were the other partici-

[62] Ibid.

[63] Quoted in Basil H. Chamberlain, *Things Japanese* (London: Kegan Paul, Trench, Trubner & Co., 1890), p. 182.

pants. They agreed that the prince should marry as soon as possible and tentatively set a date for the following May.

The date for announcing the engagement was a second major consideration, and February 11 was selected. The choice was based on the date 2,560 years earlier when Hatsukunishirasu Sumeramikoto had ascended to leadership of Yamato, near Nara and at that time the seat of governance. He was revered as the first Mikado, and was subsequently named *Jimmu Tenno* (Emperor Jimmu).

A second conference with the same participants was held on March 23, 1900, to determine whether Yoshihito's health could tolerate a marriage. All agreed that even though the crown prince was underweight, plans for the marriage should proceed. Marquis Ito Hirobumi had joined Prince Arisugawa in urging an early marriage, so that the crown prince would not have an opportunity to "touch" any other woman before the betrothal.

At a third conference on May 9, the day before the wedding ceremony, plans were reviewed and confirmed. Ito Hirobumi commented wryly on how the royal family was controlled by the court: A crown prince is "swaddled in etiquette, and when he gets a little bigger, he has to dance to the fiddling of his tutors and advisors."[64]

At this time, in recognition of his services to the emperor and his son, Baelz was invested with the Order of the Sacred Treasure, First Class. The award included an annual gift of money, which Baelz set aside as a travel fund to support his scientific and cultural pursuits.

The royal wedding was held on May 10, 1900, at the imperial palace, with the bride and groom attired in ancient Japanese court costumes. They then donned European dress for their reception at Aoyama Palace in Minato-ku. Baelz was reassured that Yoshihito stood up to the demanding ceremonies quite well. The following day he received a splendid gift of three golden sake cups, *kimpai,* from the crown prince, to commemorate his role in the wedding.

Several years later, Baelz criticized the Japanese tradition under which Yoshihito's son, Prince Michinomiya, whom he described as a lively, good-looking youngster, was taken from his parents. The child was placed under the care of Count Kawamura, an elderly admiral who was approaching seventy years of age. The parents were restricted to two visits a month, and then only for a brief period.[65]

By 1890, Erwin Baelz had completed a number of investigations on the diseases and culture of Japan. His prestige was great, and he was a man of wealth. He found himself tiring of Japan and of his situation at the medical

[64] Baelz, *Awakening Japan,* p. 124.

[65] Yoshihito was crowned as Emperor Taisho in 1912, but his mental and physical health declined steadily. Judged to be mentally incompetent in 1921, he was replaced by his son, Michinomiya, who was designated prince regent. Taisho died in 1926 and Michinomiya became Emperor Hirohito, who occupies the throne today.

school, where the professors were now convening meetings and making major decisions without consulting him. This situation reached a climax in mid-April, when commitments of which he had no knowledge were made regarding the construction of a new teaching hospital. Baelz went directly to the president (*Sori*) of the university and declared his intention to sever connections.[66] Although the president was amazed and distressed, he agreed that "the medical faculty was manifesting an inclination to run its affairs without foreign aid."[67] When the faculty members learned of Baelz's conversation with the president, they promised that he would be consulted on all future decisions and be invited to faculty meetings. Baelz was satisfied and in May retracted his notice of intended resignation.

In August 1900 Baelz left Tokyo to spend one year on leave in Europe, while Hana and Toku remained at home. He visited clinics and museums in Germany and Austria, and lectured on the cultures of the Far East. During a visit to his third brother, Robert, a leading member of the German community in London, Baelz studied the renowned Oriental collections in the British Museum.

The months of relative leisure in Europe, without the stress of his life in Tokyo, afforded Baelz an opportunity to review his future. He decided that on his return, he would withdraw from the medical faculty, complete his anthropological studes, and return for a permanent residence in Stuttgart. Therefore, within a few days of his return to Tokyo on September 3, 1901, he gave notice to the medical faculty that he did not wish to resume his work at the hospital. He also declined a new five-year contract as physician to the crown prince, but volunteered to continue informally in that role until his projected departure in early 1905.

The medical faculty held a banquet on November 22, 1901, to celebrate the twenty-fifth anniversary of Baelz's arrival in Tokyo. He described it in his diary as "the celebration of my silver wedding with the University of Tokyo."[68] Dean Ogata Masanori made the opening address and presented a handsome gold medallion to Baelz. In his response, Baelz noted that six years earlier he had proposed that he restrict his responsibilities at the school so that the Japanese could gradually take over. They had done so, and by 1902, the faculty would be 100 percent Japanese. He was confident that they were perfectly competent to continue their excellent program.

Baelz urged his Japanese colleagues to take fuller advantage of the intellectual capital that had come from the West; visiting scientists wished to sow seeds that thus far the Japanese had failed to cultivate adequately. They needed to absorb the true scientific spirit of the Western nations and to establish the special intellectual climate that this required.

His large private practice and frequent trips to such historic and scenic centers as Kyoto, Nara, and Nikko made Baelz's last years in Japan busy

[66]The first *sori* (literally, premier), Kato Hirayuki, was elected in 1887.
[67]Baelz, *Awakening Japan*, p. 123.
[68]Ibid., p. 148.

yet gratifying. He was a favorite luncheon guest of Japanese nobility and was usually the only *gaijin* (foreigner) present. He followed the events of the Russo-Japanese War closely and was pleased when Kaiser Wilhelm II openly backed the Japanese. On the Kaiser's orders, the German naval hospital in Yokohama was made available for the care of Japanese casualties; the German emperor also decorated General Nogi, the victor of Port Arthur, as a further sign of German support. Baelz's final return to Germany was scheduled for March 1905 but deferred until June so that he could accept an invitation to speak at a congress of American physicians in Manila.

The international nature of Baelz's practice was a source to him of information on many countries. In his diary entry for Sunday, April 11, 1905, he noted his opportunity to discuss world affairs with patients, including a U.S. naval surgeon, a general in the English Army, a Hindu who had studied in Edinburgh, and a Chinese medical student, who brought ". . . a letter of introduction from a German doctor in Shanghai."[69] When his office hours were finished that day, Baelz had visited a Japanese patient and at a luncheon had a long chat with a visitor from Australia.

In May came a flood of farewell dinners and luncheons given by the court physicians; by Count Arco, the German ambassador; and by the university, this last at the beautiful botanical gardens.

On June 3, Dr. Oka Genkyo, in the name of the Ministry of the Imperial Household, came to Baelz's lodgings and bestowed on him the Grand Cross of the Order of the Rising Sun. He would also receive an annual honorarium amounting to half of his annual salary from the court. Baelz described the financial award as *ashidome* (ankle irons), for he would be required to return to Japan as a consultant when called upon.

The same day, Pastor Hans Haas baptized Hana, and then she and Baelz were betrothed. He noted: "Both a little against the grain. But now that we are going home I have to take into account the conventional views on such matters."[70] On July 19, 1905, Hana and Erwin Baelz landed in Genoa and the following month set up housekeeping in Stuttgart.

Physical anthropology was one of Baelz's three favorite areas of research, and he presented his first report on the anthropological characteristics of the Japanese in a lecture at the Deutsche Gesellschaft in 1883.[71] He described them as Mongols, with yellow skin, straight black hair, a scanty beard, and an almost total absence of hair on the arms, legs, and chest. In comparison with Europeans, the Japanese had short legs and a comparatively long body, with a large prognathic skull. The height of Japanese men was about the same as that of European women, while Japanese women were proportionately smaller. Baelz emphasized the

[69] Ibid., p. 365.
[70] Ibid., p. 374.
[71] E. Baelz, "Die körperlichen Eigenschaften der Japaner," Pts. 28 and 32, *Mitteilungen der Deutschen Gesellschaft für Natur- und Volkerkunde,* 1883-84.

frequent occurrence of the so-called Mongolian spot (*Mongolenflecke*), a focal bluish gray spot, which disappeared gradually during childhood. Baelz believed that it was present only in the offspring of Mongolian peoples but later learned that it was also found in Caucasian children.

He divided the Japanese into the slenderly built, oval-faced aristocracy, and the pudding-faced *Gombei,* the farmers of rural Japan. Both groups had broad, prominent cheekbones and more or less obliquely set eyes. In comparison with Europeans, the Japanese had flat noses, coarse hair, scanty eyelashes, puffy eyelids, a sallow complexion, and short stature. The upper classes were, in his experience, often weakly.

Baelz described two historic streams of immigration into Japan. One had originated in China and flowed through Korea to the southwest coast of the main island, Honshu. A second tide had originated in Malaya and entered Kyushu through the Satsuma gateway. In his opinion, the Ainu were of quite different origin and probably were Caucasian.

At the end of September 1902, Baelz left for Hanoi to attend the Orientalist Congress and Exhibition (November 16, 1902, to February 16, 1903). It was organized by the French government, and Baelz was the delegate of the Asiatic Society of Japan, to which he had recently been elected a member. He first visited Seoul to prepare for an anthropological expedition to the north of the Korean peninsula but was recalled to Tokyo by Emperor Meiji, whose mother, *Nijo no Tsubone,* had become seriously ill.[72] In his diary Baelz explained the summons by averring that he was the only physician in whom the emperor had complete confidence.[73] His stay in Tokyo was extended owing to the illness of the crown prince, and he finally left for Indochina in November with Baron Corvisart, the French military attaché; Baron Ritter, the German attaché; and Karl Florenz, professor of literature at Tokyo University.

Because of his crowded schedule, Baelz was confined to making only brief observations on the physical anthropology of the Indochinese. He described them as being of the southern branch of the Malay race. The resemblance of the Tonkinese of Indochina to the Japanese was striking, and his Japanese colleagues were convinced that the Tonkinese were actually Japanese. Baelz believed that this resemblance supported his contention that all of the inhabitants of the countries bordering the coast-line of East Asia were closely akin. Primitive peoples from the region were present at the congress, and Baelz was especially struck by the faces of a Philippine Negrito, whom he described as "the most monkeyish creature that I have ever seen."[74]

In the middle of April 1903, Baelz returned to Korea, where he remained for three months in historical and anthropological pursuits. He

---

[72] *Tsubone* is an honorific term for a court lady of high rank.

[73] Baelz, *Awakening Japan,* p. 167.

[74] Ibid., p. 183. Negritos are the pygmies of the Far East, chiefly the Aetas of the Philippines and the Semangs of the Malay Peninsula.

investigated the graves of ancient kings and *dolmen* (the archeological term for prehistoric tombs consisting of a large, flat stone laid across upright stones).[75] The Koreans sought Baelz's advice on the origins of the bones of a bishop and two priests who had been martyred in 1843 and buried in the same coffin. Baelz promptly identified their skulls as from the Mongolian race, and noted that on one cervical vertebra there was a groove obviously made by the sword stroke that had decapitated the martyr.

Baelz extended his studies to the northern border, where there were extensive gold and diamond mines operated by the Germans. He had expected the miners to be different in their physical structure from the people of Seoul and was surprised to find that his prediction was incorrect.

The early history of Korea was of special interest to him. Near the town of Unsan, close to the Chinese border, Baelz succeeded in locating the grave of one of Korea's most powerful early monarchs.

The first in a series of quadrennial national medical congresses, interrupted only by World War II, opened in Tokyo on April 2, 1902. Taguchi Kazuyoshi was president of the meeting, but in Baelz's view the moving force was Kitasato. Baelz was a principal lecturer, and he ranged over a variety of topics. He began by emphasizing the necessity of presenting topics that would be useful to the doctors in various fields who attended from across the empire. An important aim should be an "exchange of views, and, above all, of the experiences of individual practitioners."[76] He recommended that instead of focusing narrowly on their specialty, specialists should discuss the relationship of their field to medicine and medical research as a whole.

He decried the fact that some physicians refused to divulge their therapeutic agents: "there are many doctors who practice anti-tubercular injections as a specialty, and that some of them even keep their remedies secret."[77] For Baelz, the avoidance of all noxious influences and the strengthening of the patient's powers of resistance were the essential features of effective therapy, for they gave a patient the power to cope with the bacilli. This led him to emphasize for the last time in Japan the need to strengthen the body beginning in childhood; he noted that such measures were still greatly neglected in Japan. This meant that the family doctor must watch the development of his young patients and recognize at an early age what Baelz termed "the weak spots."[78] Having recognized such defects, the physician should draw the attention of parents to them and give advice on how to protect the youth from the onset of illness. As one example, Baelz cited the fact that Japanese physicians contented themselves

[75] E. Baelz, "Dolmen und alte Königsgräber in Korea," *Zeitschrift für Ethnologie,* 1910, *42* (5): 6.

[76] Baelz, *Awakening Japan,* p. 158.

[77] Ibid.

[78] Ibid., p. 159.

with drug treatment of tuberculosis, while, he thought, they should use a preventive approach and watch for malformations of the chest that predisposed to the disease.

The importance of physical culture in preventing tuberculosis could not be overemphasized, since, in Baelz's words, it "cuts at the root of the evil."[79] In his teaching, he had always pointed out the need for an understanding by the physician of the healthy pulse, normal breathing, and normal temperature.

Baelz stressed the great importance of the practical, clinical side of medical education, in contrast to the traditional German emphasis on theoretical lectures. He had repeated this conviction throughout his twenty years in Japan and was opposed to the advocates of the theoretical and scientific philosophy. The German syllabus had recently been revised toward the practical, clinical approach to education in medicine "because it had been found that too much stress had been laid on medical 'science' whilst practical 'experience' had been ignored. Less theory, more practice! That is the watchword of the 'new syllabus.' . . . The application of knowledge is an art, not a science."[80] Japanese students, he pointed out, were already overburdened with instruction and lacked practical clinical experience.

Baelz pleaded for uniformity in the medical curricula in the three imperial universities at Tokyo, Kyoto, and Fukuoka. While the academic year at Tokyo was now divided into three instead of, as formerly, two terms, in Kyoto two terms had replaced three. Thus, in Baelz's words, "Terms, and vacations, syllabuses, and the order or examinations—all are at sixes and sevens."[81] Uniformity would allow students to move freely from university to university in the same manner as students in Germany did. In his concluding statements, Baelz lauded the history of medical education in Japan since the restoration. Medicine stood out as one of the fields in which Japan had made the greatest progress, so that Japanese names were spinkled throughout the scientific periodicals of Europe. Medical science in Japan no longer required European teachers. This state of affairs had been made possible by certain admirable aspects of the Japanese character: "great enthusiasm for a new idea; marvelous staying power and indefatigable devotion to its realization; boldness and imperturbability in the face of all privations and dangers which its pursuit entails."[82]

The last German on the medical faculty, Julius Scriba, retired in September 1901. Instead of returning to Germany, he became chief surgeon at the newly founded St. Luke's Hospital in Tsukiji, Tokyo, the year after his retirement. He had a lucrative practice and was devoted to Japan as well as to his lovely Japanese wife.

He was invited to St. Luke's by its founder, Rudolf Bolling Teussler, M.D. (1876-1934), medical missionary of the Episcopal church. Teussler

[79] Ibid.
[80] Ibid., p. 161.
[81] Ibid., p. 162.
[82] Ibid., p. 163.

graduated from the Medical College of Virginia, Richmond, and completed postgraduate studies at Bellevue Hospital in New York City.[83] He then practiced medicine in Richmond and was adjunct professor of histology, pathology, and bacteriology at the Medical College.

Although his practice prospered, Teussler was inspired to take up missionary life by the decision of his brother-in-law to become a medical missionary to China. Teussler learned of a small, unused hospital in Tokyo and wrote to the Church Missions House of the Episcopal church, seeking an appointment to Japan. Bishop McKim in Tokyo quickly accepted the young doctor. Teussler and his wife sailed from San Francisco on the *Hong Kong Maru*, bound for Kobe and Yokohama, in January 1900.

Teussler first established a small clinic in a shack on the Sumida River on the other shore from Tsukiji, at which he and a nurse-interpreter, Araki Iyo, were the entire staff.[84] Meanwhile he entered private practice in order to gather funds to purchase equipment for his hospital. In February 1902 he moved into an abandoned hospital cottage in Tsukiji to found Tsukiji Byoin, which he renamed St. Luke's International Hospital. Teussler borrowed money to build a zinc-lined operating arena for Scriba, and Erwin Baelz became the chief medical consultant.

After less than three years at St. Luke's, Scriba became fatally ill with pulmonary tuberculosis, complicated by diabetes mellitus. Seeking a change in climate, he moved to Kamakura, where he died on January 3, 1905, at the age of fifty-six.

His death came as a great loss to Erwin Baelz, who was at Scriba's bedside during his final hours. Baelz mourned deeply for an old friend and colleague of twenty-five years, and described the funeral on January 6 as an impressive ceremony with Japanese and German rituals. A battalion of Japanese soldiers in full military dress marched in the procession as a symbol of the decorations Scriba had received from the emperor: the Order of the Sacred Treasure and, posthumously, the Order of the Rising Sun. They were displayed on a cushion carried by Counts Hatfield and Metternich as representatives of the German ambassador, Count Emmerich Arco Valley. The president of Tokyo Teikoku Daigaku, Professor Dohi

[83]Howard C. Robbins and George K. MacNaught, *Dr. Rudolf Bolling Teussler: An Adventure in Christianity* (New York: Charles Scribner's Sons, 1942); *St. Luke's International Medical Center: Sixty Years of Service* (Tokyo: St. Luke's International Medical Center, undated).

[84]After the final battles between the imperial forces and the Tokugawa adherents, foreign diplomats and men of commerce thought it safer to move from Yokohama to the new capital. The Tsukiji reclaimed-land quarter was designated as the site for their homes and offices. Tsukiji developed slowly as the foreign settlement after the Meiji Restoration because the foreigners preferred the more pleasant and secure surroundings of the foreign settlements of the heights at Yokohama. Tsukiji was a mud flat whose stench was almost unbearable. The fact that it was isolated by canals on three sides and by the Sumida River on the fourth enhanced its security. Tokyo grew rapidly as the nation's capital, and foreign legations and traders felt obliged to move there. By 1872 it had become a reasonably attractive community with a significant foreign population, well laid out streets, and handsome, Western-style homes.

Keizo, and Baelz were the principal speakers; Baelz spoke on behalf of Scriba's personal friends. Pastor Haas of the Lutheran church delivered a short sermon. Count Valley then placed a wreath on the coffin in the name of the German legation, and Lehmann, doyen of the German community, placed a wreath for the Ostasiatische Gesellschaft. Baelz visited the Ministry of the Household five days later and on behalf of the Scriba family expressed gratitude for the award of the Order of the Rising Sun.

After Scriba's death, St. Luke's continued to benefit from a close relationship with the medical school, with Professors Aoyama Tanemichi, Okada Kazuichiro, Sato Sankichi, and Miura Moriharu as the chief representatives. Scriba was succeeded as head of surgery at the Tokyo Faculty of Medicine by Sato Sankichi, who specialized in thyroid surgery. One of Sato's most dramatic feats in surgery was an emergency amputation he performed on the shattered leg of Okuma Shigenobu (1838-1922), Minister of Foreign Affairs. An extremist had thrown a bomb at Okuma that shattered his leg but left him otherwise unharmed. When Erwin Baelz responded to an emergency summons, he found the minister on a sofa, with his leg "like a bag of pebbles." Sato was already on the scene and amputated immediately, with Hashimoto Tsunatsune "standing by and giving directions."[85]

In 1899, after two years of planning, Sato, Kondo, Taguchi, Uno, and Tashiro established the Japan Surgical Society. Sato was its first president, with Kondo and Tashiro as directors. At the first meeting of the society, Kondo reported two cases of gastric carcinoma on which he had performed successful surgery—he was the first Japanese to do so.[86]

Anthropology continued to be Baelz's avocation after his return to Stuttgart. Shortly after his homecoming, he spent August and September 1905 in anthropological studies at Dalmatia and the region around Trieste. The following year he continued explorations in Palestine, Egypt, and southern France. His studies on anthropology in the Far East, especially Japan, were the basis for many of the lectures that he was invited to present after his return to Germany.

In a lecture he gave in Berlin on May 19, 1906, on the prehistoric and primitive history of Japan, he postulated that the Ainu were the original Stone Age inhabitants of Japan.[87] A second population group appeared in southwest Japan during the Bronze Age and penetrated as far north as Lake Biwa, close to the present city of Kyoto. A third, and the largest, wave appeared in southwest Japan during the Iron Age and expelled the inhabitants who had settled during the Bronze Age. The new wave of

[85] Baelz, *Awakening Japan*, p. 92.

[86] Kawamata Kenji, *Igeka no rekishi* (History of Gastric Surgery) (Tokyo: Igaku Tosho Publishing Co., 1971); also *Biography of Sato Sankichi*, published by the Commemorative Society of Sato Sankichi (November 15, 1961; also *Todai Hyakunenshi*.

[87] E. Baelz, "Zur Vor- und Urgeschichte Japans," *Zeitschrift für Ethnologie*, 1907, *39* (3): 281-310.

people spread across the archipelago and by the seventh century had reached the region of present-day Tokyo. In a report to the *Zeitschrift für Ethnologie* in 1911, Baelz reasoned that the people of the Ryukyu Islands, as well as the Ainu in the north, were Caucasian and not Mongolian in their origins.[88]

Baelz had been an avid collector of the arts and handicrafts of Japan, and by the 1880s his house in Tokyo had become so crammed with woodcuts, manuscripts, embroideries, silks, wicker ware, bamboo products, and other relics that he shipped much of his collection to Stuttgart, where it was first exhibited in 1898. Ten years later he donated a large share of it to the Landesgewerbe Museum in Stuttgart, and the remainder passed to the museum (under the terms of Baelz's will) after his death. It was the most complete collection in Germany of Japanese arts and crafts.

Mental disorder continued to be one of Baelz's fields of interest. He criticized German physicians for ignoring important psychological problems. Baelz's commitment as a lifelong medical consultant to the emperor's family brought him back to Tokyo in the spring of 1908 to determine whether Crown Prince Yoshihito's health was strong enough for him to undertake a tour of Europe and the United States of America. Baelz vetoed the idea of the journey.

Once back in Stuttgart, Baelz was shaken by the news of the assassination on October 16, 1909, of his dear friend Prince Ito Hirobumi, called by many "Japan's Bismarck," and of the death of Emperor Meiji on July 30, 1912. In 1911 Baelz had become ill and diagnosed his own disorder as an aortic aneurysm, which he noted was always fatal. Death came at Neue Weinsteige on August 31, 1913.

Baelz requested that his body be autopsied and that pictures of his chest cavity be forwarded to *Jukoku* Medical Office in Tokyo; to *Kunaisho*, the Imperial Household; and to Professor Miura Moriharu of the Pathology Institute. A bequest of 3,000 Yen to Dr. Neil Cordon of Yokohama was to be used for the continuation of their joint research in the prehistory of central and south Japan. The Erwin Baelz Foundation in Tokyo received 10,000 German Marks to support Japanese doctors for studies in Germany. After the foundation terminated, the residual funds would establish the Erwin von Baelz Prize for a Japanese doctor who had done the best scientific work. Japanese students from families of low economic status would be assisted for studies in Germany through a bequest of 20,000 Marks.

[88] E. Baelz, "Die Riu Kiu Insulander, die Aino und andere Kaukäsierähnliche Reste in Ostasien," in Felix Schottlander, *Erwin von Baelz, 1849-1913: Leben und Werken eines deutschen Ärztes in Japan* (Stuttgart: Ausland und Heimat Verlage-Aktiengesellschaft, 1928), p. 159.

7

Other Physicians

It should not be assumed that the only Western physicians who taught and practiced medicine in the Meiji era were Germans. American and British physicians also played important roles in introducing Western medical practices into Japan. In addition to their other contributions, they produced a variety of informative articles on Japanese medicine.

After Britain superseded the Netherlands as the government's advisor on naval training, a British surgeon, William Anderson, F.R.C.S. (1842-1900), became the first director of the Naval Medical School in Tokyo in 1873. In his youth, Anderson debated between careers as an artist or a physician, a dichotomy of interests that characterized his life in Japan and later in London. His first aspiration was toward a career in art, and he studied at the Lambeth School of Art in London, where several renowned London artists had trained. Anderson was awarded a medal for sketching, a talent that he later applied as a teacher of anatomy; this was a practice that won the admiration of his students and colleagues. Anderson then decided to pursue a career in medicine and enrolled at St. Thomas's Hospital Medical School, London's oldest medical school, founded in A.D. 1106. Anderson's capacity for scholarship, his thoroughness, and his reticent amiability deeply impressed his teachers. He was awarded the first College Prize, the Physical Society's prize, and the coveted Cheselden Medal, named for William Cheselden (1688-1752), a distinguished teacher of anatomy and surgery at St. Thomas's. After two years as physician at the County Infirmary in Derby, Anderson returned to St. Thomas's as surgical registrar and assistant demonstrator of anatomy.

After the Meiji government founded the Naval Medical College, it looked toward the surgeons of London for a director; Anderson was the choice, in part because of his proven ability to teach both anatomy and surgery. The salary he subsequently received permitted him to marry the woman he loved, Miss Margaret Hall.

In addition to teaching anatomy, physiology, and surgery in Tokyo, Anderson served as medical officer to the British legation. The inadequate medical programs for handling venereal disease led him to recommend, in 1876, the establishment of a special program to train venerealogists. The proposal was accepted by the Japanese, and the men completing the program became effective directors of the Lock Venereal Hospital, which had heretofore been supervised by British doctors.

For an avid art student, Japan was a paradise, and Anderson took full advantage of his opportunities. He developed a varied collection of both Japanese and Chinese scrolls and other art forms, pottery, and lacquer ware.

After his return to London in 1886, Anderson rejoined the staff at St. Thomas's as joint lecturer in anatomy and assistant surgeon. He was advanced in 1891 to the position of surgeon and also took over direction of the section on diseases of the skin.

Meanwhile, Anderson continued in his enjoyment of Japanese and Chinese art and in 1866 published *The Pictorial Arts of Japan.* He donated his collection to the British Museum and with Ernest Satow as co-author published the *Descriptive and Historical Catalogue of Japanese and Chinese Paintings in the British Museum.* It presents a complete history, based on painstaking research done together with Satow on the religions, superstitions, and literature of art treasures of Japan and China.

Several Japanese students, attracted in large measure by Anderson, came to St. Thomas's to learn medicine; the most distinguished was Takagi Kanehiro (also Kenkan).

Anderson died suddenly in 1900. For his role in naval medical training he was posthumously awarded the Order of the Rising Sun, Third Class. His collection of Japanese and Chinese art in the British Museum shares a place with the treasures that Engelbert Kaempfer brought to Europe from Japan two centuries earlier, in 1693.

After one year as a missionary at Kanagawa, Duane B. Simmons, M.D. (1834-1889), resigned and started on a rewarding medical career in Yokohama. As one of the best surgeons in the rapidly growing port city, he developed a large consulting practice, derived from both the foreign community and from referrals by native physicians. After seven lucrative years in Yokohama, Simmons returned to New York City in 1868, where he practiced for a single year before going back to Japan. He was then appointed chief surgeon at the Yokohama Shichu Byoin (Yokohama City Center Hospital), founded in July 1872 by the governor of Kanagawa Prefecture. In the same year a new facility was erected and the name changed to Yokohama Kyoritsu Byoin, with Matsuyama Toan as director. In February 1874, the name was changed to Juzen Byoin. Simmons also served as advisor on public health to the government in Tokyo.

Simmons enjoyed writing and produced some of the most informative descriptions of disease problems and medical practice in Japan. In an article in the *China Imperial Customs Report,* 1880, Simmons joined other physicians in attributing *kakke* to a specific exhalation from the soil, primarily in the low-lying towns on the eastern and southern shores of the islands.[1]

---

[1] D. B. Simmons, "Beriberi or the 'kak'ke' of Japan," *China Imperial Customs Medical Report* XIX, 38 (Shanghai, 1879-80).

The following year, he published a description of the major disease problems.[2] Simmons stated that the absence of reliable governmental mortality records was attributable to the sharply limited diagnostic ability of over 90 percent of Japanese practitioners.

The highest mortality was among infants, which Simmons ascribed in part to inefficient or an entire absence of medical treatment. He cited as the leading causes of infant death diarrhea, cholera infantum (an often fatal, noncontagious childhood diarrhea of the summer months), and especially "affections of the nervous system terminating in convulsions." These nervous affections he accounted for on the basis of the Japanese custom of shaving the heads of infants in the first year of life: "tied on the backs of nurses or their elder brothers or sisters, [they] are often exposed to the rays of the sun quite unprotected by any kind of covering."[3] A fatal form of capillary bronchitis and other respiratory disorders were, in Simmons's view, also attributable to the exposed shaven heads.

Simmons disagreed with Erwin Baelz, who had reported eight cases of scarlet fever. If it existed, he maintained, Baelz was the only physician who had observed it.

In his role as sanitary advisor to the government during the severe smallpox epidemic of 1875, Simmons succeeded in having a system adopted for control of the epidemic, as well as for the prevention of future outbreaks. A system of house-to-house inspection was instituted, and all victims were removed to a hospital or cared for by physicians specifically designated for such duties. Vaccination was compulsory for individuals who had not been vaccinated or had not suffered from the disease. And, because all citizens were registered by their municipality, only a few were able to avoid the program. Since Simmons's system had been adopted, there had been no cases of smallpox in Yokohama.

The control of leprosy was attributed by Simmons to the Japanese belief that it was hereditary. As a result, marriage was not approved until both families had been assured that there was no history of the disease in the other. Simmons was impressed with the health status of children who lived with their families in the foreign settlements: "[These] may, in fact, be regarded as an asylum of safety for children, as in the space of six years I have in my own practice lost but two children, and those in a weakly family."[4]

In another communication to the *Medical Record*, January 1882, Simmons made a series of wide-ranging comments on Japan.[5] In regard to the climate, he believed that because of its mild and equable nature it was unsurpassed in the world, yet it was debilitating to most foreign residents

---

[2] D. B. Simmons, "The diseases of Japan," *Medical Record,* 1881, *19:* 90-92.
[3] Ibid., p. 90.
[4] Ibid., p. 91.
[5] D. B. Simmons, "Medical notes on Eastern and Southern Asia," *Medical Record,* 1882, *21:* 248-49.

because of the long summer heat and mild winters. The air, which was always moist, lacked "that bracing quality necessary for healthful invigoration and recuperation."[6]

The adverse effects of the climate were most pronounced in women, especially pregnant ones. They were not able to nurse their infants for longer than three to four months, and even then, milk flow was insufficient, so that artificial feeding was essential. Convalescence from confinement was protracted; uterine discharge was prolonged and recurred on exertion.

Both mother's milk and that of Japanese cows produced colic, indigestion, and diarrhea; Simmons preferred imported condensed milk with barley, oatmeal, or rice water. Japanese mothers used malt diluted with water or water from rice that had been boiled for a long period as a substitute for milk.

Simmons ascribed postpartum fever to a "puerperal malarial fever," which at times was accompanied by profuse uterine hemorrhage. He treated most of his postpartum patients with quinine during the first fortnight.

Simmons joined other Western physicians in disparaging the indigenous system of medicine.[7] Although Western-style medicine had made remarkable progress since the opening of the country, about 79 percent of the practitioners still used the traditional system, and he predicted that they would continue to do so for many years. He attributed this to the fact that "the government requires no qualification of those who have been in practice up to the present time. . . . By far the greatest portion of these are the merest pretenders and quacks of the worst sort, ignorant often not only of the Chinese characters in which the medical books are written but of their own written language."[8] In the case of a protracted illness, patients were usually treated by a succession of practitioners with whom the association was so transient that the patients did not know their doctors' names. On the other hand, for a mild ailment the neighborhood pharmacist served as the medical adviser.

The tradition of restricting a physician's fee to the sale of medication kept most traditional practitioners in the rural areas, and some in the cities, close to penury. Their fee usually amounted to no more than four to six cents a day. Because of the added costs, medications were never dispensed as tinctures, which would require bottles and corks. Instead, pills, powders, and little packages of roots and herbs were made by the patients into infusions. By another cost-saving practice, pills and ointments were dispensed in small clam shells instead of boxes.

Practitioners of Western-style medicine had abandoned the day-charge system and required a fee for each prescription. Yet patients would pay only a consultation fee to foreign doctors, and as far as Western-style

⁶Ibid., p. 249.

⁷D. B. Simmons, "Medical practice in Japan, old and new," *Medical Record*, 1881, *19*: 204-6.

⁸Ibid., p. 204.

Japanese physicians were concerned, "Well-to-do and grateful patients . . . usually present their doctor with small sums of money, but more often this gratuity consists of a box of eggs, a fowl, or a small piece of silk or cloth."[9]

The emperor's health status was evaluated daily. Every morning, one or more of Tokyo's leading practitioners came to the palace and meticulously took the *Tenno's* pulse, using the traditional Chinese techniques.

A disagreeable medical custom was the filthy condition allowed to the patients. They were not washed during an illness—even to the extent of cleansing the teeth or washing the face, fingers, nails, hair, or beard. (Western-trained practitioners who insisted on having their patients bathed were dismissed.) A beneficial therapeutic measure was the requirement that patients were permitted to drink only water that had been heated. In the case of a severe illness, their diet was restricted to soft-boiled rice diluted with water; Simmons suggested that for this reason many patients died from inanition rather than from disease itself.[10]

Japanese practitioners trained in Western medicine continued to prescribe mercury for syphilis: "So universal has it been the custom of the disciples of the old school of medicine in Japan to use mercury in the treatment of all venereal sores that, in nearly twenty years of hospital and private practice among the natives, I have rarely met with one who ever had a chancre who has not been thoroughly mercurialized by stuffing the nostrils with cotton or paper saturated with the drug."[11]

Simmons commented on the absence of puerperal fever. He had never seen a case of the infection and attributed this to the tradition of propping the mother after delivery on her knees, with a group of pillows behind her back for support. This encouraged the flow of lochia, thereby preventing the invasion of infectious organisms.

Simmons did not share Erwin Baelz's enthusiasm for hot mineral springs. In his view, they did as much harm as good.

Simmons also commented on the use of moxa and acupuncture. The latter, he thought, was beneficial in the relief of painful neuralgia because if a nerve sheath was punctured accidentally, the pressure from accumulated serum was relieved.[12] He was aware of two patients who had serious problems because the slender needles had penetrated the spinal membranes between the cervical vertebrae.

The Chinese Maritime Customs Service posted a physician in each of the seventeen treaty ports under its jurisdiction. They reported to R. Alexander Jamieson, M.D., the medical director, who was also editor of the *Chinese Customs Medical Reports.* The publication was an invaluable source of information on medical and sanitary problems and progress in

[9] Ibid., p. 205.
[10] Ibid.
[11] Ibid.
[12] Ibid., p. 206.

the Orient. It also included selected communications from authors who were not connected with the Customs Service.

The official duties of the medical officers of the treaty ports included medical care of the staff and of a ship's personnel when no surgeon was aboard, and free care to indigent Chinese. They were also required to conduct sanitary inspection of all ships calling at their ports. They performed many other duties. For example, Patrick Manson conducted meteorological observations at Amoy. In 1870 all of the medical officers, save one Chinese, were British. During his return passage to America in 1822, Simmons combined information from the Customs Reports with some from other sources.[13] He included information on a range of medical problems in the major treaty ports, beginning with opium smoking, which at that time was a major concern to the English Parliament.

Simmons had discussed the problem with respectable Chinese practitioners, who told him about an asylum for addicts in Peking. It was supported by voluntary subscriptions and by the sale of a pill of secret ingredients that was said to relieve addiction. Opium smoking was widespread in all classes and was increasing steadily, especially among the affluent. In Simmons's words, "A pipe of opium is to the Chinese host what a glass of sherry is to the Western gentleman, and is offered to guests in the same way—as a sign of hospitality. In a word, opium smoking is in China what dram drinking is in England and America, no more nor . . . less."[14]

Simmons postulated that opium smoking was less harmful than addiction to alcohol, since the opium addict was harmless while the alcoholic was belligerent and destructive. He attributed the severe emaciation of the opium addict to malnutrition and starvation rather than to any specific effects of the drug.

Dr. P.B.C. Ayres, colonial surgeon in Hong Kong, found that sudden and complete withdrawal from long-standing addiction was not as traumatic as was often predicted. From this study he concluded that reports of the evil effects of opium smoking were much exaggerated. In another study, he tested addicts with three samples: from one he extracted all morphine; the second, a 7½ percent solution, was the customary opiate; while a third contained a double dose, 15 percent opium. The addicts reported that all three were equally good, a finding that Ayres could not explain. He shared the opinion of other medical men of the East, that opium eating was a far greater danger than smoking.

Shanghai, with the largest foreign community, had a debilitating climate and a foul water supply. There were only eleven Western physicians, of whom the largest number were Irish, and five hospitals—four for Chinese and one for foreigners. Simmons attributed the low mortality in the foreign

---

[13]D. B. Simmons, "Medical and sanitary notes on the foreign settlements of Eastern and Southern Asia," *Medical Record,* 1882, *21:* 386-88.

[14]Ibid., p. 387.

settlements to the custom of going to Japan or to a health resort on the coast of North China in the case of illness.

The health and medical situation in humid, semitropical Hong Kong was mixed, with 5,000 foreigners and 250,000 Chinese. The four hospitals included one governmental, one civil, one lock, and one for Chinese. The latter had been built and still served as a "dying house," a place where Chinese could succumb, since families did not wish to have anyone expire in the home. To avert such an event, they would go to the extreme of putting a dying person out on the street.

Surgical care in Hong Kong was "something horrible to witness. In fact, the cases . . . are often assisted to die, by the use of thoroughly irrational and barbarous means."[15] This perplexed Simmons because although the Chinese were said to have faith in Western surgeons, they scrupulously avoided them.

Saigon, a French colony, was said to be extremely unhealthy. The mortality from all disease in the colony of Singapore, on the other hand, had dropped by one-half since British public-health programs had been established. While cholera and typhus were major problems in nearby Java, cases in Singapore were rare, probably because of the excellent aqueduct water supply. A cholera epidemic that was just abating in Java had resulted in two to three thousand deaths during a period of three months, a mortality rate of 80 to 90 percent. Because of the outbreak, Simmons had not been able to visit Batavia, where the epidemic had been most severe.

Duane Simmons returned to the United States in 1882, his health impaired, and lived in New York City and Poughkeepsie. He studied Japanese history and in 1886 published an article on leprosy in Japan.[16] The same year, he returned to Japan to complete his research and died there in 1889.

The first American physician to go to Japan, James Curtis Hepburn (1815-1911), was also a pioneer in other fields: he was the compiler of the first English-Japanese dictionary; the inventor of the system of writing Japanese in Roman letters, *Romaji;* and the first to translate the Bible into Japanese. A medical missionary of the Presbyterian Board of Foreign Missions, Hepburn was a strict Calvinist, endowed with warm, humanitarian instincts.

Born into a devout Presbyterian family at Milton, Pennsylvania, in 1815, Hepburn followed the Presbyterian collegiate trail to Princeton, where he graduated in 1832. For his medical studies he chose the University of Pennsylvania and was awarded the doctorate in medicine in 1836. After five years of practice, he entered the mission field in March 1841 and with his wife, Clarissa Lette Hepburn, was assigned to China. During four

---

[15] Ibid.

[16] D. B. Simmons, "Leprosy in Japan," *Transactions of the Medical Society* 21 (Syracuse: 1886): 448-54.

frustrating years in Amoy, their first three children died. Hepburn mastered Chinese, Malay, and Japanese, which were to prove invaluable for his future work in Japan.

From China, Hepburn returned to Manhattan in 1846, where he practiced ophthalmology for thirteen years. The success of the Perry expedition rekindled his interest in the Orient, and he sailed for Japan under the banner of the Presbyterian church. He studied Japanese grammar and the Gospel of St. John on the hundred-day voyage from New York to Hong Kong, whence he sailed to Shanghai and arrived at Kanagawa on October 17, 1859.

A section of a decrepit and abandoned Buddhist temple, Jobutsuji, in Kanagawa on the Tokaido, was made available at a rental fee of six dollars per month for Hepburn to use as his home and clinic. There he sat, at a table in a ten-by-twelve-foot room, three times a week, but visited by no more than a handful of patients. He found the people to be courteous and friendly, while the government was "feudal and jealous of foreigners."[17] Before each session of his clinic, Hepburn read to his patients from the Holy Scriptures.

His consuming dedication was to the study of Japanese, and he began to prepare for his monumental English-Japanese dictionary and the translation of the Bible. After four months, his only medical consultations had been with his own countrymen, save for a single Japanese patient. Despite the dangers facing foreigners in Japan, Hepburn was fearless in responding to calls for his medical services. On January 6, 1860, he rode a horse fifteen miles through samurai country to prescribe for Consul Townsend Harris.

After a year and a half, in April 1861, the local authorities assented to his request for permission to rent a temple on the Tokaido in Kanagawa for a dispensary and a hospital.[18] The majority of his patients had ophthalmic problems, and by May 17, he was seeing fifteen to twenty patients a day. Two Japanese studied medicine and English. Meanwhile, Mrs. Hepburn, an intelligent and energetic lady, and as equally endowed with humanitarian attitudes as her husband, taught classes in English.

By July 11, 1861, the number of dispensary patients had risen to 100 or 150, some coming from long distances. After five months, Hepburn had performed a total of thirty-one operations for pterygium, entropion, cataract, and one enucleation.

The fact that Hepburn was teaching Christian doctrine along the most traveled thoroughfare in Japan, in the face of longstanding harsh interdicts against Christianity, was responsible for the termination of the clinic at Kanagawa. In September 1861 he was ordered to close his program there and move to the foreign quarter at Yokohama.[19] Here he continued to combine the practice of medicine and surgery with the dissemination of

[17]Letter, October 20, 1959.
[18]Letter, April 17, 1861.
[19]Letter, September 8, 1861.

Christian doctrine. In December 1862, the *Bakufu* asked Hepburn to teach English, geometry, and chemistry to nine young men: "Japanese officials came and requested it . . . agreed to my stipulation. My heart failed me but I could not retreat . . . . If you knew how hard it is to drill these hard and rigid mouths into emitting correct English sounds."[20]

Within one year of their move to Yokohama, Mrs. Hepburn made a pathbreaking step for the education of women in Japan, when she opened the first school for females. The well-known Ferris School for Girls of the Reformed Church of America grew out of Mrs. Hepburn's school. With her warm hospitality, she made the Hepburn home in Yokohama a haven for American naval officers. Dr. Hepburn's surgical reputation extended to Edo, and on April 13, 1864, he reported that six doctors from there had brought him difficult cases.[21] In the Fifth Annual Report of the Mission, in 1864, Hepburn was described as being "widely and favorably known amongst the people, and frequently consulted by native physicians."[22]

Japanese students of medicine as well as practitioners came to Hepburn's clinic to learn Western practices and techniques.[23] One year later, his popularity had grown even more, and he was performing many operations each day, largely ophthalmological.[24]

One of Hepburn's more memorable surgical feats was the amputation of a leg of the famed Kabuki actor Sawamura Tanosuke, and the subsequent application of a prosthesis from America, said to be the first Western prosthesis used in Japan. In March 1865, Hepburn reported that he had amputated the arm of a Japanese soldier, the first amputation ever performed on a Japanese and observed by doctors as well as students.[25]

The following year, 1865, Dr. Hepburn established the Yokohama Academy, where he taught English and the Bible to classes of forty students each. And, as a diligent corresponding member of the American Geographical and Statistical Society, he systematically recorded meteorological observations.

Up to Hepburn's time, the only semblance of an English-Japanese dictionary was the handwritten *Ageria Gorin,* by an unknown author (1814). Hepburn published the first complete English-Japanese dictionary, *Waei Gorin Shusei,* printed at the Presbyterian Mission Press in Shanghai in 1867.[26] He spent several months at the press supervising the printing and

[20] Letter, December 9, 1862.
[21] Letter, April 13, 1864.
[22] D. Thompson, *Fifth Annual Report,* October 3, 1864.
[23] Letter, April 25, 1865.
[24] Letter, June 2, 1866.
[25] Letter, March 16, 1865.
[26] An incomplete Portuguese-Japanese dictionary had been circulated in 1603, and several efforts were made in the eighteenth century to prepare Dutch-Japanese dictionaries. Early in that century, a Nagasaki interpreter, Nishi Zenzaburo, started to compile a dictionary based on Peter Marin's Dutch-French dictionary, *Woordenboek der Nederduitsche*

reading the proofs. Along with the dictionary, he introduced his invaluable *Romaji* system, which greatly facilitated communication by making it possible to convert Japanese characters into the Roman alphabet. John R. Black, a leading foreign journalist living in Yokohama, who tended to be critical of Americans, lauded Hepburn's achievement. "Hepburn," wrote Black, "had done more than any other toward opening the door of knowledge to the people of Japan."[27]

Hepburn continued to work on his masterpiece, and while the first edition was only 132 pages, the second, published five years later, in 1872, also in Shanghai, contained 900 pages. He added Chinese characters with numerous phrases and sentences as examples of their usage. An abridged version was published in New York in 1873, and by 1907 it had been through fifteen editions.

The first translations of the Scriptures to an Oriental tongue were completed by Robert Morrison (1782-1834), at Macao. As a theology student, Morrison had chosen the missionary life and opted for China. To prepare himself for the field, he walked the wards at St. Bartholomew's Hospital Medical School in London in 1805 and learned the rudiments of astronomy at Greenwich. He also studied with a Chinese tutor. After his ordination by the Scots Church in January 1807, with an appointment to the London Missionary Society, Morrison sailed for Macao, where he arrived the following September. In 1810 he published a translation of the Acts of the Apostles, and on November 25, 1819, he completed an entire version of the Old and New Testaments. His mastery of the Chinese language encouraged him to prepare a dictionary, which was published in Macao under the patronage of the Honorable East India Company in 1817. The company attached such importance to Morrison's dictionary that they brought from England a press and a printer.[28]

Because Japan was closed to the West, missionaries, primarily under the auspices of British faiths, concentrated their efforts along the South China coast. One of them, Reverend Charles Gutzlaff, who was sent by the Netherlands Missionary Society, made the first translation of the Scriptures

---

Fransche taalen: Dictionnaire flamand et français (Amsterdam and Utrecht, 1729), but he never finished the task. Aoki Konyo in 1758 prepared an incomplete Dutch-Japanese lexicon on the orders of the Tokugawa shogun Yoshimune. Inamura Sanpaku, a student of *Rangaku*, with several assistants completed *Haruma wage*, a Dutch-Japanese dictionary of 80,000 words, in 1796. It was too massive for publication. The most widely used Dutch-Japanese dictionary, *Nagasaki* or *Dofu Haruma*, based in part on François Halma's *Nieuw Nederduitsch en Fransch Woordenboek* (Amsterdam, 1717), was prepared by the distinguished *opperhoofd* Hendrik Doeff, during the idle months when trade between Batavia and Nagasaki was suspended by the Napoleonic Wars.

[27]John R. Black, *Young Japan* (London, New York: Oxford University Press, 1968), p. 73.

[28]Lindsey Ride, *Robert Morrison: The Scholar and the Man* (Hong Kong: Hong Kong University Press, 1957), p. 13.

into Japanese. With the assistance of a shipwrecked Japanese sailor, he translated the Gospel according to St. John and the Acts of the Apostles into *Katakana.*[29]

At about the same time, S. Wells Williams, L.L.D., of the American Legation in Peking, with the help of another shipwrecked Japanese sailor translated the book of Genesis. It was never published.

The next effort was that of Reverend D. Bruno Bettelheim, M.D., of Hungarian-Jewish origins, who was serving in the *Lew Chew* (Ryukyu Islands). Beginning in 1845, he translated the four gospels and the Acts into the *Lew Chew* language. They were revised to the Japanese idiom and sold to the British and Foreign Bible Society, under whose auspices they were published in *Hiragana* in Vienna in 1872.

After the publication of his dictionary in 1867, Hepburn embarked on the translation of the Scriptures into *Romaji.* He began with a Bible tract, *A True Doctrine Explained,* written in Chinese by D. Bethune McCartee, M.D., a Presbyterian medical missionary in Ningpo. Cut in secrecy, in wooden blocks in Yokohama and smuggled to Shanghai for printing, it was the first Christian tract published in the Japanese empire. Hepburn led a translation committee consisting of Reverend D. C. Greene, D. D., L.L.D., the first missionary sent to Japan by the American Board of Commissioners of Foreign Missions, and Reverend Samuel R. Brown, who had come to Nagasaki with Verbeck in 1859. They were assisted by four Japanese. The complete translations of the New Testament into the Japanese vernacular were published in 1880, as *The New Testament in Japanese,* transliterated by J. C. Hepburn, Yokohama, *Seishi Bunsha,* 1880. To celebrate the grand occasion, on April 19, 1880, representatives of fourteen missionary societies gathered in the Christian church in Tokyo. The translation of the Old Testament was completed and published in 1887.

In 1887 Hepburn was elected president and professor of physiology and hygiene at Meiji Gakuin, a Christian university founded in Tokyo in 1886 by the U.S. Presbyterian church, Scottish Presbyterian missions, and the Dutch Reformed Church. It represented a merger of Tokyo Icchi Shin Gakko, established in 1877 by Icchi Kyokai, a Japanese Christian; Tokyo Icchi Eiwa Gakko, founded at Tsukiji in 1883; *Daigakko,* which had started as Hepburn *Juku;* and Yokohama Senshi Gakko. Subsequently, Hepburn gave personal funds to the school for the construction of a student dormitory.

A Bible Dictionary, completed by Hepburn in 1891, enabled the Japanese to understand the message and the meaning of events recorded in the Scriptures. His friend and devoted biographer, W. E. Griffis, described this task as "perhaps the literary work which Dr. Hepburn most enjoyed personally, and at which he wrought with minutely loving care."[30]

[29]This work was published by the press of the American Board of Foreign Missions in Singapore in 1838.

[30]William Elliot Griffis, *Hepburn of Japan and His Wife and Helpmates* (Philadelphia: The Westminster Press, 1913), p. 157.

After thirty-three years in Japan, Hepburn retired at the age of seventy-seven, and returned to America in October 1892. He settled in East Orange, New Jersey, and on his ninetieth birthday Ambassador Takahira came there from Washington to present the Third Order of Merit of the Rising Sun and the decree of appointment. His greatest American honor came in the same year, when his alma mater, Princeton University, also recognized his remarkable contributions in Japan. Saluted as the oldest living graduate of Princeton, Hepburn received an honorary doctorate of laws, with the following accolade: "venerated scholar, translator, physician, and herald of the Cross in the Far East."[31]

John Cultery Berry, M.D., a medical missionary from Philadelphia, could be described as a universal man. He made major contributions to medical care and education, nursing training, and health education in an extended region centered at Kobe. He was as well the pioneer of prison reform on a national level; and as a dedicated missionary, at every opportunity he combined the word of God with his medical tasks.

After graduating from Jefferson Medical College in 1870, Berry became the first medical missionary of the American Board of Commissioners for Foreign Missions to go to Japan. He arrived in Kobe, which had become the rapidly expanding seaport for Osaka, with a budding foreign population in 1872. It had been opened for foreign residence in January 1868. Berry was assigned to be director of the International Hospital in Kobe and received as remuneration a ward for his Japanese patients and an examining room.

Berry gained the goodwill of the Japanese practitioners by inviting them to accompany their patients when they referred them for consultations. Thus the practitioners had no reason to worry about losing their patients; they collected the customary fee and as a dividend gained new information about diagnosis and therapy. Moreover, since Berry explained his findings and recommendations to the accompanying physician, he could be sure that they were understood and carried out, and thus the chances of a successful therapeusis were significantly enhanced.

After ten months, ten Japanese youths began to study the rudiments of medicine with Berry, and in the winter of 1872-73, he petitioned the prefectural authorities for permission to perform autopsies for his students on the unclaimed bodies of criminals. The request was forwarded to Tokyo, where it was approved with the additional prerequisite that the local authorities construct a proper dissecting room for Dr. Berry's use. It was completed in May 1873, but owing to his other responsibilities, Berry did not have an opportunity to put the new facility to use until the following November. The first dissection, in that month, performed on two corpses, was a comprehensive teaching exercise that attracted physicians from the adjoining community, Hyogo, and the surrounding prefectures. A brief history of anatomy based on the introductory lectures of his former teacher

[31] Ibid., p. 213.

at Jefferson, W. W. Keen, M.D. (1837-1932), a neurosurgical pioneer, was read in Japanese for one and a half hours. Regular instruction in anatomy began the following day, with some fifty students; Dr. Thornicraft, a British practitioner from Kobe, served as Berry's assistant. Shortly thereafter, a Japanese physician assisted in teaching anatomy, which was based on translations of chapters of Keen's edition of *Heath's Practical Anatomy.* Another Japanese, Dr. Kimura, was responsible for teaching chemistry and physiology. Berry lectured on materia medica, surgery, the theory and practice of medicine, midwifery, and gynecology.

In the meantime, Berry expanded his efforts to Himeji, a historic castle town thirty-four miles southwest of Kobe, where he established a hospital with forty beds. Under his supervision a network of six dispensaries opened within a radius of twenty miles of Kobe, and each month Berry attended a total of from five hundred to seven hundred patients. Since Hepburn was an eye specialist, the Japanese assumed that because Berry was an American doctor he must be skilled in the same field: "The result was large clinics of eye diseases at my clinic and hospital from the very first."[32]

In the communities where his dispensaries were established, Berry developed what may have been the first organized program of continuing education for practicing physicians in Japan. He met with Japanese practitioners on each visit to the network of dispensaries and in addition to practical demonstrations discussed instructional papers that he had prepared and circulated before his visit. The papers presented didactic principles, which he based on his Philadelphia lecture notes; he prepared them daily and sent them to the nearest dispensary for further transmittal around the network. As W. W. Keen noted when he read a paper of Berry's in Philadelphia: "In this way about 120 native physicians who could not leave their school for purposes of study were taught the most important elementary principles of the science."[33] Berry usually focused his papers on immediate problems, such as outbreaks of smallpox and cholera.

By 1879 Berry's consultative network extended to Okayama, eighty-nine miles from Kobe, where he also taught medicine. From the beginning, his success as a practitioner was attributable in part to his policy that the more affluent citizens should pay for the medicines dispensed to the poor. By February 1874, this plan was working so admirably that in addition to paying for medicines, the affluent had raised $2,500 for the construction of three charitable infirmaries.

Education of the public on the problems of health and hygiene was another project of John Berry's. He used Kobe newspapers for articles on infant and child health, housing, sanitary practices, and other preventive measures.

---

[32]Quoted in Griffis, *Hepburn of Japan,* p. 124.
[33]W. W. Keen, "On medical missionary works with some notes on the condition of medicine in Japan," *Transactions of the College of Physicians and Surgeons,* 3rd ser. vol. 4 (Philadelphia, 1879), pp. 15-16.

John Berry was the pioneer in bringing about the reform of the Japanese prisons, which at the time epitomized inhumanity. His interest was stirred when one of his students was appointed physician to a prison and described to Berry the abysmal state of affairs. The student reported that hygiene and sanitation were virtually nonexistent; drinking water was foul and often unobtainable besides. Ventilation was inadequate, and no effort was made to rehabilitate the prisoners. *Kakke* was rife.

In October 1873 Berry sent to the authorities in Kobe a report on the state of the prison where his students practiced. He volunteered to inspect all prisons in Japan and to make recommendations on their improvement. Based on his findings, they included (1) need for a central authority over prisons; (2) categorization of all prisons; (3) special training courses for prison officers; (4) instruction of prisoners in trades and home industries; (5) establishment of prisoners'-aid societies; (6) abolition of corporal punishment save for the most violent crimes; (7) opportunity for continuing communication between a prisoner and his family; (8) introduction of hygienic and sanitary practices; (9) adequate care of the sick; and (10) teaching Christianity as an agent for the reform of prisoners.[34]

The government acknowledged Berry's report with gratitude and distributed it to all prisons as the directive to reform.

The Japanese continued to loathe lepers, and those sufferers who could not support themselves because of physical deformities, such as loss of fingers and toes, were cast out to die on the streets as vagrants. Berry shared the common belief that leprosy was an inherited disease and pointed out that its incidence could be limited to no more than five generations if its victims received proper care. He recommended that since no specific curative agent had been discovered, the emphasis should be on hygienic, medicinal, and moral therapy.

For the eradication of leprosy, Berry recommended the enactment of a law requiring (1) lepers to restrict marriage to other lepers and of the same generation through five successive generations; (2) establishment of a major national leprosarium in a locality with a moderate climate; (3) investigation of the sanitary factors that favor or are adverse to the appearance of leprosy; (4) supervision of lepers by the government with isolation in proper leprosaria; (5) appointment of physicians-in-residence to manage such institutions; and (6) public education on leprosy. When he returned to America in 1877 because of illness, Berry stated that the central government had committed itself to cooperation on implementing his recommendations.

John Berry was also the motive force in the introduction of modern nursing training in Japan. It began with the founding of Doshisha ("single purpose association") University, the first Christian university in Japan, in Kyoto in 1875 by Joseph Hardy Neejima (also Jo Niijima) (1843-1890).

[34]Ibid., pp. 16-17.

Born on Hokkaido, Niijima was interested in the United States from his youth. He was trained and educated to serve as a writer and tutor for his master, Prince Itakura. When he requested permission to study English, the prince ordered him to pursue studies of the Dutch language instead, but Niijima pored over an English Bible in secret.

During the summer of 1864, he decided to flee from Japan and seek an education in the United States. With the help of a local shipping clerk, Niijima persuaded Captain William Savory of the American brig *Berlin*, anchored at Hakodate, to take him to Shanghai. There he was allowed to board the *Wild Rover*, commanded by Captain Horace Taylor and owned by the Alpheus Hardy Company of Boston.[35] On the long passage to New England, Niijima, who had been dubbed "Joe" by Captain Taylor, studied English intensively. But as is true of most Japanese, speaking English was far more difficult for him than reading it.

The *Wild Rover* dropped anchor in Boston in August 1865, and Niijima was assigned to the Sailor's Home. Here he was asked to write an explanation of his flight from Japan. The earnestness of his statement made such an impression on Alpheus Hardy that the shipowner decided to defray the costs of the young man's education. After two preparatory years at Phillips Academy in Andover, Massachusetts, Niijima enrolled at Amherst, where he received a B.S. degree in 1870 and, having converted to Christianity, began the study of theology. The following year the government of Japan granted him official permission to remain in the United States to complete his studies. Although he had been corresponding with his family secretly, he could now write to them openly.

When the special mission under Iwakura Tomomi, minister of foreign affairs, visited America in early 1872, Tanaka Fujimaro from *Mombusho* studied the organization and practices of education. Niijima accepted an invitation to serve as advisor and interpreter for the mission. When their studies in America were completed, he accompanied the mission to Europe in May 1872 and served as secretary to Tanaka.

Niijima was ordained into the Congregational ministry on September 24, 1874, and arrived in Japan as a missionary of the American Board of Commissioners of Foreign Missions in December of the same year. The interdicts against evangelistic work by Christian missionaries still applied, and in 1875 Niijima established a center for Christian training in Kyoto, which became Doshisha University. The center was restricted to male students for the first two years, after which females were also permitted to enroll.

Niijima envisaged a medical school in association with his university and as the first step established Doshisha University Hospital. As general director of the hospital, Berry sent an appeal to the Women's Board of

---

[35] Arthur Sherburne Hardy, *Life and Letters of Joseph Hardy Neesima* (Boston and New York: Houghton Mifflin and Co., 1891). See also *Daijimmei Jiten*, vol. 5 (Tokyo: Heibon-sha, 1962), p. 51; and *Sekai Daihyakka Jiten*, vol. 23 (Tokyo: Heibon-sha, 1972), p. 215.

Missions in Boston, Massachusetts, for financial support in developing the hospital and establishing an associated school of nursing at Doshisha.[36]

The first program in nurses training was opened at Yushi-kyoritsu-Tokyo Byoin in April 1885 by Dr. Takagi Kanehiro, with Miss M. E. Reed as director.[37] Planning for the program had been initiated in October 1884. The second program was established by John Berry at Doshisha University, in the autumn of 1886.

In 1885 the Women' Board obtained the services of Miss Linda Richards, who was the first professional nurse in America. Having served as the head of the Massachusetts General Hospital Training School and of the Nurses School at the Boston City Hospital, she possessed an eminently useful training for her new task in Japan.

Melinda (Linda) Ann Judson Richards (1841-1930) was attracted to a career in nursing by the desperate need for nurses during the Civil War.[38] She left the factory in Foxboro, Massachusetts, where she was employed and became an assistant nurse at the Boston City Hospital. But she could foresee little if any opportunity for learning nursing skills there and registered at a school opened by Dr. Susan Dimock at the New England Hospital for Women in Boston. After one year, she was awarded a diploma and then spent a year at Bellevue Training School in New York, the first American nursing school modeled on the Nightingale system. Richards returned to Boston as superintendent of the Boston Training School, which later became the Massachusetts General Hospital School of Nursing. She was then made responsible for opening a nurses' training program at the Boston City Hospital; it was the first nurses-training program developed as an integral part of a hospital.

When Richards arrived at Doshisha, the physical plant included a nurses' dormitory, a general ward, and a maternity ward.[39] Berry, as medical director, was assisted by Dr. Sarah C. Buckley, physician and gynecologist; a young Japanese Christian, Dr. Shirafuji Nobuyoshi, taught anatomy, physiology, and hygiene. There were five nursing students enrolled for a

[36]Before the appearance of training schools for nurses, nursing practices either at a hospital or in the home had not existed. As Linda Richards, the founding director of the program in Kyoto, noted: "If a member of the family was for any cause taken to a hospital, the other members of the family went in turn to stay with and care for him, and it was from their own trained nurses that the Japanese learned the necessity of better care for the sick." Linda Richards, "Nursing progress in Japan," *American Journal of Nursing,* April 1902, 2 (7): 492. Miss Richards went on to note: "The primary object in establishing training schools for nurses in Japan was to provide for young women an additional profession by means of which they could become self-supporting and at the same time maintain their social position and dignity." Ibid., p. 493.

[37]Ishihara Akira, *Kango Shi* (Tokyo: Igaku Shoin Ltd., 1971).

[38]Linda Richards, *Reminiscences of Linda Richards: America's First Trained Nurse* (Boston: Whitcomb and Barrows, 1911); Edward T. James, ed., *Notable American Women, 1607-1950* (Cambridge, Mass.: The Belknap Press, 1971), vol. 3, pp. 148-50.

[39]*The First Annual Report of the Doshisha Hospital and Training School for Nurses* (Kyoto: The A.B.C.F.M. Mission, April 1887).

period of two years, with the first month to be spent on probation status. Linda Richards gave instructions on nursing; Dr. Buckley lectured on anatomy, physiology, and hygiene. English-language nursing texts that had been translated into Japanese were used for teaching. The lectures were followed by practical work on the wards. Daily prayer services for the nursing students were also attended by in- and outpatients.

A total of sixteen inpatients had been admitted, seven of whom were diagnosed as suffering from eye disorders, mainly conjunctivitis and trachoma. Almost half of the patients in the outpatient clinic were also classified as eye cases.

Berry expressed concern over the primitive facilities provided for Linda Richards, and lauded her tolerance of the situation:

In the want of a house, the superintendent of the school has been put to a very trying inconvenience, and, coming from an institution where, in her work, she should command all that wealth and organization could effect, it is certainly to her credit that she has borne, as she has, the privations and inconveniences to which our necessities have subjected her. To allow this condition of things to continue, however, is fatal to our work and in the highest degree unjust to her.[40]

The rules and regulations of the school, published in April 1887, stipulated that the most desirable age for admission was thirty to forty years; candidates were required to be able to read Scriptures, to write legibly, and to be "quick and careful" in observation. Tuition was free, and uniforms were furnished by the school. The curriculum extended over two years; the student was on a probationary status for the first month. Courses included nursing, anatomy, hygiene and physiology, and the Holy Scriptures.

Strict regulations governed the nurses' dormitory; students were required to be in the building by 9:00 P.M., and all the lights were to be out with no talking or laughing permitted after 10:00 P.M. Guests were restricted to the parlor, and students were not permitted to have guests in their rooms. No visitors were allowed on Sunday.

The religious emphasis was also prominent in the rules governing the hospital. In addition to the medical staff, there was to be an evangelist: "It shall be his first duty to contribute to the spiritual welfare of the patients. . . . He shall hold morning and evening prayers. . . . He shall be present in the waiting-room during the out-patient service, and shall hold private religious conversation with such as may show an interest in the Truth. . . ."[41]

After deliberating for several months, Linda Richards decided that the school should adopt the traditional uniform of American nurses—a blue striped gingham dress with a white apron and bib and a white muslin cap.

[40]Ibid., p. 5.
[41]"Rules and Regulations, Doshisha Hospital, Kyoto Training School for Nurses. Established and conducted in connection with the A.B.C.F.M. Mission. Rules, Requirements, and Curriculum of Study." (Yokohama: R. Meiklejohn & Co., April 1887).

In deference to Japanese custom and for purposes of economy, quiet, and comfort, she permitted her students to wear conventional Japanese straw sandals.

The patient load grew steadily, and in his Sixth Annual Report, March 31, 1892, Berry reported a total of 200 inpatients and 2,199 outpatients, with 123 surgical procedures.[42] Eye cases constituted 29 percent of all outpatients; digestive disorders, 22 percent; and respiratory, 12 percent.

Berry led a medical-nursing evangelistic mission to Ogaki after a devastating earthquake that took place there on October 28, 1891. The team included four doctors, three nurses, and a clergyman; they had to obtain official endorsement from the government before they set out from Tokyo. Berry reported on the carnage: "The injuries treated were of exceptional severity. Fractures, dislocations, and flesh wounds predominated. These latter were especially severe about the head, face, and back, and having, in most cases, received no attention were in a filthy and dangerous condition."[43] He paid tribute to the conduct of the Japanese, both the injured and those who had been spared: "Kindness and sympathy characterized the attentions of the well to the injured. . . . The patient submission of the injured, their courage in suffering, and their confidence in and appreciation of the services rendered contributed much toward sustaining the members of the different corps in the difficult performance of their work."[44]

Ten nurses graduated in June 1892, all of them Christians.

In reporting on his medical activities, Berry commented on his striking success in treating *kakke* patients by means of a rice-free diet. He had successfully treated several cases of heart involvement from *kakke* using sodium salicylate, spirits of ether nitrate, and strophanthus. He reported that he had abandoned Koch's procedure for the treatment of tuberculosis with tuberculin, since all of his patients had in this way become progressively worse.

In his final report, in 1893, Berry described the value of the branch dispensary that the hospital had opened in a poor section in Kyoto.[45] A program of training in district nursing for the final-year students afforded them an opportunity to care for patients in their homes. The hospital had opened a mission infirmary known as "The Sanatorium," to provide medical care for missionary workers in the interior of Japan.

Since the work of the nurses in many instances paralleled that of a physician, a modified Hippocratic Oath was developed to be taken as a public pledge at the time of graduation:

[42] *The Sixth Annual Report of the Doshisha Mission Hospital and Training School for Nurses* (Kyoto, 1892).

[43] Ibid., p. 5.

[44] Ibid., pp. 5-6.

[45] *The Seventh Annual Report of the Doshisha Mission Hospital and Training School for Nurses,* Kyoto, in connection with the Japan Mission of the American Board. For one year ending March 31, 1893 (Tokyo: Seishi-Bunsha, 1893).

The Nurse's Pledge

1. I hereby solemnly affirm that to the best of my ability and judgment, I will use the knowledge which I have gained in the art of caring for the sick and suffering only for the benefit of my fellow-men and the alleviation of distress.

2. That I will, in all my relations with the sick and afflicted, make their interests and their recovery my chief concern.

3. That I will under no circumstances make public any secret which may be to the detriment of any person or persons, a knowledge of which I have obtained through my professional intercourse with them.

4. And that I will, in all particulars, conduct myself so far as lies in my power in such a manner that I shall in no way bring reproach upon the noble profession which I now enter, but will seek to honor it by an upright life and sincere devotion to the duties devolving upon me.

Signed_____[46]

Berry left Japan permanently in 1893. His experience in handling eye diseases in Japan and his association with Hepburn led him to postgraduate studies in that field in Vienna. He then practiced opthalmology and spent his final years in Worcester, Massachusetts.

At the first graduation ceremony, on June 26, 1888, four young women received their diplomas; seven diplomas were awarded in 1889, and six in 1890. Richards returned to America soon after the 1890 graduation ceremony. Unfortunately, after 1896, misunderstandings between the Mission Board and Doshisha led to withdrawal of the hospital and training school from the university.

Fifteen years after she founded the school in Kyoto, Linda Richards was pleased with the improved position of women in Japan and the role that nursing had played in it. Richards wrote: "Japanese women have . . . come forward to stand side by side with women of other nations, and in this progressive movement the nursing profession has proved no insignificant factor."[47] She was convinced that nursing education in Japan was at the same high level as in the Western world: "This question is often asked: 'Are the Japanese nurses who are trained in their own schools as well and thoroughly instructed as nurses in schools in other countries?' Surely they are, is the reply which we are most happy to give."[48]

The development of the northern island, Hokkaido, as an agricultural resource, a new frontier, and a defensive post against Russian settlements in the Kuriles was an early goal of the Meiji government. A new department, *Kaitakushi* ("pioneer mission"), referred to as the Hokkaido Colonization Office, was established for the development of Hokkaido.[49] Kuroda

---

[46]Ibid., p. 8.

[47]L. Richards, "Nursing progress in Japan," p. 491.

[48]Ibid., p. 493.

[49]The most important contribution of the Hokkaido Colonization Office was the founding of the Imperial College of Agriculture at Sapporo by William Smith Clark, Ph.D. (1826-1886), president of the Massachusetts Agricultural College at Amherst, Massachusetts.

Kiyotaka, deputy commissioner of the department, came to America in early 1871 to enlist the services of specialists as advisors to the program because of the American experience in large-scale farming. He also wished to purchase machinery and equipment for the enterprise and to arrange opportunities for Japanese to study agricultural and mechanical programs. With the help of Mori Arinori, the first Japanese resident minister in Washington, Kuroda had the good fortune to secure the services of General Horace C. Capron (1804-1885) of the U.S. Army, who was the first U.S. Commissioner of Agriculture under President Ulysses S. Grant. After a brilliant record in the Civil War, Capron turned his considerable energies to agricultural projects and developed large-scale farms in Maryland and Illinois.

The Capron mission arrived in Japan on August 22, 1871, with a staff of eight men, including agricultural specialists, engineers, and geologists. It included as well a young physician, Stuart Eldridge (1843-1901), who had been serving as a librarian for the Department of Agriculture. Eldridge was born in Philadelphia and served with the Wisconsin Regiment in the Civil War. He graduated in medicine at Georgetown and was an instructor in anatomy when he joined the Agriculture Department to help organize a library. When Eldridge went to Hokkaido in 1872 with the team of field workers from the Capron mission, in addition to his own routine tasks he taught anatomy at Hakodate Medical Institute, which opened in August 1872. In July 1873, the school had a total enrollment of seventeen students. In 1874 Eldridge's lectures were translated by Honda Kimitoshi and published in three sections as *Kinsei Isetsu* (modern medical theory). He also taught and cared for patients at the City Hospital. Continuing frustration and antagonism were rife among the members of the mission, and when Eldridge's contract expired in November 1874, he decided not to renew it.

Stuart Eldridge decided, though, to remain in Japan and the following year opened a practice in Yokohama, where he was to remain for twenty-seven years. He became medical director of the imperial hospital; he was also the chief surgeon of the Foreign General Hospital of Yokohama. Hygiene and public health were a second area of interest for him, and he was advisor to the local hygiene department as well as to the American consulate. In 1883, Eldridge also became a member of the staff at the Central Hygiene Office.

Despite his manifold activities, Eldridge wrote a variety of articles about diseases and medicine in Japan, which he published in Japan and

---

Clark graduated from Amherst in 1848 and earned a Ph.D. in botany and chemistry at Göttingen in 1852. Clark came to Japan in 1876 and in 1876-77 founded the Agricultural College at Sapporo. Owing to his strong New England Christian convictions, Clark combined Christian instruction with his lectures; he refused to teach a class in ethics unless he was permitted to teach the Bible at the same time. At his departure from Sapporo in 1877, Clark's devoted students asked him for a farewell message; his words, "Boys, be ambitious!" became an enduring slogan for Japanese youth.

America. On December 20, 1883, Eldridge, then medical director of the Imperial Hospital of Kanagawa Prefecture and surgeon in charge of the Foreign General Hospital of Yokohama, wrote a perceptive analysis of the state of Japanese medicine.[50] He began by commenting that he wished to correct the fallacious notion held by many residents of foreign countries that Japan was an Eldorado replete with the overflowing wealth of the Orient. In actual fact, save for a small and rapidly dwindling number of government employees, foreign practitioners worked harder and for even less remuneration than did practitioners in smaller cities in America. Furthermore, the cost of living in decent comfort was far higher in Japan than in the U.S. These financial strictures were compounded by a severe financial crisis; business was at a standstill, and since foreign practitioners derived their income from the foreign community, they were in serious financial straits. Their plight was also attributable to the continuing reliance of the Japanese on native physicians to whom, save for occasional modest gifts of cash, remuneration was solely in the purchase of medications.

In the larger cities, such as Osaka, Kyoto, Kobe, and Tokyo, the Japanese could consult foreign physicians employed by government hospitals, to whom they were not required to pay a fee. On the other hand, these physicians were being replaced rapidly by Japanese who had studied medicine in Europe and by graduates of the medical faculty in Tokyo. Eldridge noted that the foreign physicians such as himself were in less demand: "for Japan has, perhaps, made more real and solid progress in medical science than in any other branch of western learning and now has a considerable number of fairly good men either educated in foreign countries, where some have won honors, or under foreign instructors in the Government hospitals and medical schools at home."[51] In almost every town of the empire there was at least one Japanese practitioner who had some understanding of Western medicine.

A further incentive to change was the government's encouragement of the advancement of Japanese practitioners in medical science, and appointments to government medical posts were available only to those with an understanding of Western medicine. Furthermore, in regard to private practitioners, "a system of examination and graduated license has been put in force throughout the Empire, which would afford no bad model for adoption in some of the United States."[52]

Eldridge lauded the rapidly advancing program for the publication of medical literature. Some 400 medical texts had been forwarded to the Surgeon General's Library in Washington; many were beautiful reproductions of American and European originals, while others were Japanese texts displaying equally excellent craftsmanship. An equal number of texts

[50]Stuart Eldridge, "The present state of medicine in Japan," to the editor of the *Medical News,* Philadelphia, January 26, 1884, *44:* 112-55.

[51]Ibid., p. 112.

[52]Ibid.

would be sent to Washington in the near future, and full sets of Japanese medical journals were also available to American readers.

As a surgeon, Eldridge was naturally interested in the quality of surgical instruments manufactured in Japan, and he found them to be indistinguishable from the best imported products. The sole area of inferiority was in the production of small steel products, and he anticipated that this would be remedied in the near future.

While remarkable progress had been made in most areas of medicine, anatomy was still in a backward state: "Though Japan has an anatomy law, which many of our benighted States would do well to copy, its operation is so hampered by the prejudice and mistaken benevolence of the people that even in the great city of Tokio (Yedo) the Imperial School of Medicine is unable fully to supply its students with anatomical material, while in the provincial hospitals and schools opportunities for dissection are rare indeed."[53] Therefore, teaching of anatomy relied primarily on elaborate atlases, wall plates, and reproductions of Auzoux's papier-mâché mannequins.

Eldridge found the Japanese admirably suited to perform operative surgery: "Steady nerve, marvelous dexterity, mechanical tact, and a power of mentally reconstructing form that is absolutely astonishing are qualifications to which, if a knowledge of anatomy were added, the product should be a surgeon above the average."[54]

In Eldridge's view the slavish adoption of German medical education was inappropriate to the intellectual capacities and the needs of the Japanese. He based this contention on his experience that "quick, ready, and intelligent as the Japanese undoubtedly are, their mental calibre is, in many respects, that of precocious children, and their science is, and for a considerable period must remain, imitative and routine."[55] Eldridge felt that the objective at the Tokyo medical school "to turn out men fitted for original investigation of the deepest mysteries of science and versed in all the theories of modern medicine proved or purely hypothetical" was misguided, when Japan's urgent need was for physicians to deal with the everyday diseases of the country.[56] Instead, the handful of graduates who had been able to withstand the stress of the German program at Tokyo practiced therapeutic nihilism, and the welfare of the patient was completely subordinate to the doctor's interest in the natural history of the disease. This attitude was even more evident in the students than in the teachers.

Japanese students actually preferred to be taught in the English language and to use American and English texts. However, the government had imposed the German political system as being more in accord with the

[53] Ibid., p. 113.
[54] Ibid.
[55] Ibid.
[56] Ibid.

Japanese culture than the free thought and institutions that characterized English-speaking peoples.

Plants, minerals, and animal substances continued to be an important part of indigenous medicine. Each year cargoes of dried fetal deer were shipped from Hokkaido to Honshu and Kyushu and to China. Dried lizards, tiger claws and teeth, bear bile, monkey skulls, and more repulsive substances were widely used.

Eldridge paid tribute to the advances in Japanese obstetrics wrought by Kagawa Shigen, who had developed the field to a parity with European obstetrics of a century earlier. Yet Kagawa had unfortunately clung to the Japanese tradition of secrecy and refused to divulge his innovations to other physicians.

Eldridge closed his communication by describing the therapeutic value of an extract of malt known in Japan as *mizuame*. He described it as a clear, transparent, faintly brown or amber-colored syrup that, if water were not added, had the consistency of candy. It was a mixture of malt and starch that, owing to the presence of malt, caused the starch to ferment to a saccharine substance, maltose. Until recently the use of *mizuame* had been as an easily digestible and fortifying food for the aged and for handfed or weakly infants. Eldridge was probably the first Western physician to call attention to the merit of *mizuame,* which had been used for centuries in cases of dyspepsia and gastrointestinal malfunction.[57] Now it was used widely for these disorders by foreign practitioners, and it was far more effective than pepsin or artificial gastric juice. He hoped that it would be given a thorough trial in America "without the clap-trap and advertising falsehood which repel every honest physician."[58]

Eldridge discussed the high incidence of aortic aneurysm in the European population in Japan at a meeting of the Society of Alumni of Bellevue Hospital on December 6, 1893, during a home leave that he took in order to regain his health.[59]

In Yokohama, with its average population of 2,000 to 2,500 Europeans, statistics for 1871-77 showed that deaths from aneurysm were exceeded only by those from tuberculosis and smallpox. He noted that deaths from tuberculosis were almost invariably among recent arrivals. Many deaths listed as "heart failure" or "hemorrhage" were, in Eldridge's opinion, probably due to aneurysm. He himself had in nineteen years cared for some forty Europeans who died from aneurysm, and he reckoned that there was an average of five deaths per year. An equal frequency was observed by his friend and colleague in Yokohama Dr. Edwin Wheeler, also an American.

[57] In 1881, in a communication on the diseases of Japan, D. B. Simmons, discussing the use of malt as a milk substitute, stated: "Malt has been used from time immemorial by the Japanese for various forms of dyspepsia and weak digestion."

[58] S. Eldridge, "The present state of medicine in Japan," p. 115.

[59] Stuart Eldridge, "Occurrence of internal aneurysm in European residents of Japan," *New York Medical Journal,* February 10, 1894, *59:* 165-68.

The upper part of the thoracic aorta was most frequently involved, followed in order by the lower part, and then the abdominal aorta. Eldridge emphasized that he had seen only four cases of aneurysm involving other major vessels.

The course was a rapid one, with early rupture. Thus, even though the existence of an aneurysm was readily evident to an experienced practitioner, surgical intervention was not possible, since the site could not be determined before the patient's demise.

Longstanding advanced syphilis was cited as the etiological factor, and the disease almost exclusively afflicted long-term residents. Since their wives did not usually accompany them to Japan, the Europeans often took Japanese mistresses, who were usually not infected. But the men who strayed to the arms of common prostitutes, whom Eldridge termed "the frail sisterhood," often contracted syphilis.[60] In a survey in 1868, George Newton, an English physician, had shown the incidence of the disease in the "sisterhood" to be in excess of 90 percent.

Secondary factors in the tissue degeneration leading to aneurysm were, in Eldridge's view, high living and heavy drinking, both of which were rife among European males enjoying the bachelor life.

While aneurysm, characteristic of advanced syphilis, was frequently seen in the European community, it was uncommon among the Japanese. Eldridge believed that if an ethnic group such as the Japanese suffered from syphilis for centuries, "they developed a relative tolerance by inheritance."[61] Thus the serious advanced lesions did not appear. Since untreated syphilis had been a universal infection for centuries in the lower strata of Japanese people, their tolerance was high. He cited as a comparable example the experience during the Peninsular Wars, 1808-14, when Wellington's army was almost decimated by a spirochete to which they had not been previously exposed. On the other hand, Iberian soldiery had no problems, since for centuries they had been exposed to the strain.

Eldridge postulated the existence of an unknown factor, which he believed was filariasis, but so far he had searched in vain for filarial lesions in the aneurysmal area. However, such studies were limited in Japan by the fact that autopsies were extremely difficult to obtain. Wheeler, on the other hand, believed that malaria was the unknown factor.

The treatment of syphilis in Japan had improved strikingly because of the five or six thousand younger Japanese practicing physicians who had been educated in modern scientific medicine and surgery at Tokyo University and in Europe. Eldridge concluded by advising his fellow physicians to warn patients planning to visit Japan that governmental prophylactic programs for the brothels were, as elsewhere, largely ineffectual. Furthermore, "Clandestine prostitution, at least in the open ports, has increased *pari passu* with the stringency of discipline in the regular army of Venus,

[60] Ibid., p. 167.
[61] Ibid.

and there are few parts of the world more dangerous to the unsophisticated globe trotter than fascinating, childlike, beautiful, glorious *Dai Nippon.*"[62]

In the discussion, Dr. Albert L. Gihon, who had served as senior medical officer on the hospital ship U.S.S. *Idaho,* stationed in Nagasaki, confirmed Eldridge's statement about syphilis in Japan. Gihon was convinced "that it was at the bottom of all the other diseases [he had] encountered there; this made the practice of medicine comparatively simple."[63] Gihon also commented on the proclivity of Japanese practitioners to be overzealous in administering mercury and potassium iodide in treating syphilitic patients: "With their accustomed haste and lack of thoroughness [they] went to work and very generously salivated their countrymen."[64]

Eldridge returned to Japan in 1895 with his health restored, and resumed the practice of medicine. In 1900 he was elected vice-president of Seiikai (medical society), founded by Takagi Kanehiro and his associates in May 1881. Eldridge died on November 16, 1901, in Yokohama and was posthumously awarded the Order of the Sacred Treasure, Third Class.

The first medical-training program in Kyoto was established at Shoren-in Temple, Higashiyama, by M. Makimura, governor of the prefecture, in 1872.[65] Junker von Langegg, a German who was a British subject, was invited to direct the program, and he assumed the responsibilities in August of that year. His first clinic was in a *ryokan* (Japanese inn) in north Kyoto. In November of the same year, Langegg moved his program to Shorenin. Langegg was a dismal failure as a teacher; his arrogance turned both the students and the other teachers against him. When his contract expired in September 1875, its renewal was opposed, and he was reappointed on a temporary basis for only a three-month period.

G. C. Mansvelt, who was teaching at Kumamoto, came to Kyoto as Langegg's successor in May 1876 but grew frustrated at the prefectural government's opposition to changes in the program that he considered essential. After one year, Mansvelt moved to the National Training Hospital in Osaka, where he remained until 1879.

Heinrich Botho Scheube (1853-1923) came to Kyoto as Mansvelt's successor in October 1877. Scheube had spent his youth in Greiz, Upper Saxony, where he was born on August 18, 1853. He graduated in medicine at the University of Leipzig in 1875. After several months in Vienna, Scheube returned to Leipzig, where he served as the last assistant to the renowned Karl Wunderlich.

Scheube was not only an excellent teacher and physician but as well a productive scholar of medicine and Japanese culture. He used his summer

---

[62] Ibid.; p. 168.

[63] Ibid.

[64] Ibid.

[65] It became the Kyoto Prefectural College of Medicine, which is today the only prefectural medical school in Japan. From 1944 to 1951, the school added a Women's Medical College, which closed when medical education in Japan became coeducational.

holidays for field trips across Japan and in 1880 studied the Ainu on Hokkaido. He described them as hairy, squat, filthy, and addicted to drunkenness.[66] Their religion, he wrote, deified nature: the sun, the wind, the ocean, and especially the bear. At a meeting of the Deutsche Gesellschaft in 1880, Scheube presented an extensive description of the Ainus as a bear cult.[67] He identified the bear as their deity, whom they acclaimed by worshipping carved pieces of wood. They sacrificed the animal with an extensive ritual and devoured the meat in a fervent religious rite.

Scheube shared Erwin Baelz's theory that *kakke* was an infectious disease.[68] To support this position, he pointed out that even the most affluent families had not been immune to an epidemic that he studied in Kyoto and Tokyo in 1881. He was also interested in age distribution and found that in the same epidemic fewer than 6 percent of the cases in Kyoto were children. An analysis of 993 cases in Tokyo showed that 80 percent were in the fifteen-to-thirty-years age group; 15 percent, between ten and fifteen years; and the remainder, over thirty years of age.

Scheube was probably the first person to show that *kakke* was a disease of the peripheral nerves. By histological investigations, he demonstrated degeneration of the nerve fibers, which drew the following comment in 1882 from his friend Erwin Baelz: "Scheube has conducted detailed and exhaustive studies on all clinical and histological aspects of the disease."[69]

Scheube was a dedicated clinician as well as a scholar and spent long hours at the hospital, arriving at 8:00 A.M. and frequently not leaving until midnight. Because of the continued reluctance of Japanese women to be examined by a male, he saw three times as many men as women in his polyclinic. In his hospital wards the ratio was even higher: four men to one woman. According to Japanese tradition, post mortem examinations continued to be opposed in Kyoto, and only a handful were performed during Scheube's four years in Japan.

When the staff of the medical school and hospital (called Kyoto Igakko) decided in July 1880 to move to a new site on the west bank of the Kamo River at Hirokoji, Kawaramachi, Kamikyo-ku, Scheube introduced European design for the new buildings. In 1903, *Mombusho* granted the school the status of an Igakko Senmon Gakko (medical technical college).[70]

In the beginning of May 1882, Scheube left Japan for an extended homeward journey, during which he conducted medical and ethnographic studies in China, Siam, Singapore, Java, and Ceylon. From his studies in

[66] H. B. Scheube, *Die Ainos* (Yokohama, 1882).

[67] H. B. Scheube, "The bear cult and bear festivals of the Ainu with several remarks about their dances," *Mitteilungen der Deutschen Gesellschaft für Natur- und Volkerkunde*, 1880, *21:* 44-52.

[68] H. B. Scheube, "Die japanische Kak'ke," *Mitteilungen der Deutschen Gesellschaft für Natur- und Volkerkunde*, 1880, *28:* 170-74.

[69] Erwin Baelz, "Über das Verhältnis der multiplen peripherischen Neuritis zur Beriberi (*Pannauritis endemica*)," *Bulletin Hirschwald* 1881-1883, in *Zeitschrift für klinische Medizin*, 1882, *4:* 616-17.

[70] See *Nihon Rekishi Daijiten*, vol. 6 (Tokyo: Kawade-shobo, 1964), p. 94.

Japan and his observations on the trip, he wrote *Die Krankheiten der waermen Laender* (4th ed., Jena: 1910). It went through four editions and was translated into several languages. In it, as in all other aspects of his career, Scheube demonstrated scrupulous attention to detail and an infinite capacity for hard work.

He resumed his career as a lecturer at Leipzig in January 1883, but after two years returned to his ancestral home in Greiz to become director of the National Hospital. His final post was as senior public-health officer in his native Greiz, where he died February 2, 1923, at the age of seventy.

T. W. Beukema spent fifteen years as a physician-surgeon and teacher in Tokyo, Yokohama, Osaka, and Nagasaki. Born June 10, 1830, he studied medicine at Utrecht from 1855 to 1859; Antonius Bauduin was one of his teachers. At graduation, he became medical officer, third class, in the Netherlands army. After earning a doctorate in medicine in Groningen, Beukema studied medicine in Berlin and France under military auspices and on his return taught at the Army Medical School in Amsterdam. In 1871, Beukema was invited to join the staff of the Osaka Army Hospital as a Dutch army officer, and he assumed these new responsibilities the following year. He also served at the Army Hospital in Tokyo until he retired from the Dutch Military Medical Corps in 1877. Beukema then spent three years, 1877-80, on the staff of the Tokyo Government Hospital, after which he served for a similar period at the Yokohama Juzen Hospital. Beukema was also elected to the Japan Central Public Hygiene Society.

The Nagasaki Medical School and Hospital were the site of Beukema's final posts in Japan; he was the last Hollander to join the staff, where he practiced and taught from March 1883 to December 1887. Beukema was succeeded by an English physician, Charles Arthur Arnold (1862-94). Arnold left the medical school in a few years and opened a private clinic in Nagasaki, where he practiced until his death in 1894.

8

Epilogue: The Meeting of the Twain

The phenomenon of the rise of Western medicine in Japan is, we have suggested, without parallel in world history. There stood in its way such obstacles as the country's rigidly enforced isolation, including harsh governmental decrees against all Western contacts; a special and fierce vigilance against Christianity; and an everlasting language barrier.

The two systems of medicine that came into confrontation were fundamentally divergent. For a millennium, the Japanese practiced traditional Chinese medicine, *Chung-i,* which was completely nonscientific. Under that system, a complete knowledge of the structure and function of the human body was impossible to obtain, because dissection was banned. Western medicine, by contrast, began to expand its scientific base starting with Andreas Vesalius (1514-1564) and his first reliable human dissection (1543), and with William Harvey (1578-1657) and his discovery of the circulation of the blood.

At the time when the "twain" first met, medicine was virtually ignored. The Portuguese, as the first Westerners to establish an association with the Japanese, had little to offer in that area. The Iberian peninsula was isolated from such advances in medicine as were taking place in the city states of northern Italy and the Netherlands. Furthermore, no physician ever figured prominently in the Portuguese missions in Japan.

Circumstances changed sharply after the arrival of the Dutch, for a medical man was almost always an essential member of their staff at Dejima. The Dutch doctors were quite willing to teach medicine: some did so partly because they enjoyed it and partly in order to learn about Japan, while others viewed giving instruction in medicine merely as an outlet to relieve the boredom of their life at Dejima. The status of the Dutch outpost as a medical-training center during its first fifty years was enhanced by the presence of several gifted doctors, such as Daniel Busch, Willem Ten Rhijne, and Engelbert Kaempfer. The opportunity for physicians from Germany and Sweden to serve there brought leading medical scholars to Japan.

Since a vast materia medica was a central pillar of Chinese medicine, the information that the Japanese sought at Dejima had primarily to do with Western therapeusis. Two factors strengthened this interest: the zeal of the Japanese for medication and self-medication, and the popularity of medicines as a Dutch imported commodity. The "final bow" of the Dutch, the establishment at Nagasaki of the first Western medical school in the Orient, was a fitting farewell.

Beginning with the Meiji Restoration, the Japanese embarked on a course of intensive borrowing and adapting from the West those programs in technology and science that seemed best-suited to carry Japan rapidly to world prestige. In making those appropriations, the Japanese slavishly copied German medicine, not only because of its position of world leadership, but also because they found its philosophy and style especially comfortable. Emerging slowly from more than three centuries of feudalism, the Japanese discovered that their German teachers came from a similar social order; a form of feudalism was in fact the basis of the organization of the faculty and its relationships with the students in the German universities.

The Germans' strong emphasis on fundamental research as opposed to the study of the patient also appealed to the Japanese. As members of a family-centered society with a tradition of *ongi,* or lifelong obligation for a favor bestowed, Japanese physicians were less willing than were their Western counterparts to establish compassionate doctor-patient relationships. This disinclination became an inherent part of the imperial-university system: a professor was dedicated to his research laboratory, and instruction of the student at the bedside held a decidedly secondary position.*

Some minor differences distinguished the two approaches. While German students moved freely from medical school to medical school, Japanese students remained at one institution throughout the medical course. Also, a unique relationship between medical schools evolved in Japan. Tokyo Imperial University Faculty of Medicine controlled faculty appointments and promotions in the schools in the Kanto region and the northwestern half of Japan. The faculty members in those institutions were graduates of Tokyo, and all aspired to return there one day as professors. A similar "satellite" relationship characterized Kyoto Imperial University Faculty of Medicine and the schools of southwest Japan, beginning at the Kansai region and including the Japanese medical school in Mukden, Manchuria.

Japan's final choice in medicine lay between the German and the English systems, the first being a research-oriented approach and the second, one that stressed care of the patient and teaching at the bedside. The decision, as we have seen, was for German medicine. Perhaps the Japanese would have developed a more rounded medical education if they had combined the two: the German emphasis on research throughout the curriculum, linked with the English pattern of strong patient-oriented teaching in the clinical years.

---

*This pattern did not prevail in the *senmon-gakko,* or second-level medical schools, where research was minimal and the emphasis was on turning out practitioners. During the *semmon-gakko* period, patients preferred those graduates to ones from the imperial universities, because the attitude of the former was more humane.

In taking the unusual step of recommending to the Berlin government that Prussian military medical officers rather than university professors be sent to Tokyo, the German ambassador Brandt probably made a sound decision, yet it might have gone awry if the government's choice had not been Leopold Mueller, who could be called an ideal person for starting a medical school. Even so, Mueller is a relatively "unsung" hero in comparison with Erwin Baelz, the leading physician in Japan after the Meiji Restoration.

The dominance of the Germans at Tokyo overshadows the work of doctors from other countries. Such men as William Willis and J. C. Hepburn, who labored under more hazardous circumstances than did the Germans, also facilitated the fusion of Eastern and Western medicine in Japan. Still, their impact was minimal compared with that of the Germans, whose style was so suited to Japanese culture that it prevails even today.

Bibliography

In this bibliography some of the Japanese authors have abided by the traditional custom of putting their surnames first; others have reversed the procedure by Anglicizing their names.

Achiwa Goro, M. D. "Linda Richards in Japan." *American Journal of Nursing,* August 1968, *68:* 1716-19.

Alcock, Sir Rutherford. *The Capital of the Tycoon: A Narrative of a Three Years' Residence in Japan.* 2 vols. London: Longman, Green, Longman, 1863.

Anderson, William, F.R.C.S. "On art in its relation to anatomy." *The British Medical Journal,* 10 August 1895, *ii:* 349-58.

"William Anderson, F.R.C.S." *St. Thomas's Hospital Gazette,* November 1900, *10:* 171-73.

Artelt, D. W. "Die Grundung und die ersten Jahrzehnte der Berliner Medizinischen Fakultät." *Ciba Zeitschrift,* 1956, *7:* 2570-2605.

Baelz, Erwin. *Awakening Japan: The Diary of a German Doctor: Erwin Baelz.* Edited by his son, Toku Baelz. Translated from the German by Eden and Cedar Paul. New York: The Viking Press, 1932.

_____ . "Die körperlichen Eigenschaften der Japaner." *Mitteilungen der Deutschen Gesellschaft für Natur- und Völkerkunde Ostasiens,* 1883, *31:* 330-59.

_____ . *Lehrbuch der Innerenmedizin mit besonderer Rücksicht auf Japan bearbeitet.* Tokyo: Verlag von T. Kanahara, 1900-1901.

_____ . "Dolmen und alte Königsgräber in Korea." *Zeitschrift für Ethnologie,* 1910, *42* (5): 776-81.

_____ . "Über die in Japan vorkommenden Infektionskrankheiten." *Mitteilungen der Deutschen Gesellschaft für Natur- und Völkerkunde Ostasiens,* 1882, *2* (27): 295-319.

_____ . "Über japanisches Familienleben." *Chronik aus Schwabischer Merkur,* 19 and 22 July, 1893.

_____ . "Über permanente Thermalbäder." *Berliner klinische Wochenschrift,* 1884, *21:* 765.

_____ . "Prehistoric Japan." *Smithsonian Institution Annual Report of the Board of Regents,* 1907, 523-47.

Bartholomew, James R. "Japanese Modernization and the Imperial Universities, 1876-1920," *Journal of Asian Studies,* February 1978, *37:* 251-71.

_____ . *The Acculturation of Science in Japan: Kitasato Shibasaburo and the Japanese Bacteriological Community, 1885-1920.* Ann Arbor, Michigan: University Microfilms, 1972.

Barus, Elinor and James A., eds. *Naval Surgeon: Revolt in Japan 1868-1869. The Diary of Samuel Pellman Boyer.* Bloomington, Indiana: Indiana University Press, 1963.

Beasley, W. G. *The Meiji Restoration.* Stanford, California: Stanford University Press, 1972.

Beauchamp, Edward R. "Griffis in Japan: The Fukui Interlude, 1871." *Monumenta Nipponica,* 1975, *30* (4): 423-52.

Berry, John C. *Medical Work in Japan.* Boston, Mass.: Women's Board of Missions, Congregational House, 1872.

Black, John R. *Young Japan. Yokohama and Yedo. A Narrative of the Settlement and the City from the Signing of the Treaties in 1858 to the Close of the Year 1879. With a Glance at the Progress of Japan during a Period of Twenty-One Years.* 2 vols. 1883. Reprint. London, New York: Oxford University Press, 1968.

Borton, Hugh. *Japan's Modern Century.* 2nd ed. New York: The Ronald Press Co., 1970.

————. *Peasant Uprisings in Japan in the Tokugawa Period.* New York: Paragon, 1968.

Bowers, John Z., M. D. *Medical Education in Japan.* New York: Harper & Row, 1965.

————. *Western Medical Pioneers in Feudal Japan.* Baltimore and London: The Johns Hopkins Press, 1970.

————. "The adoption of German medicine in Japan: The decision and the beginning," *Bulletin of the History of Medicine,* 1979, *53:* pp. 57-80.

Boxer, C. R. *The Dutch Seaborne Empire, 1600-1800.* New York: Alfred A. Knopf, 1965.

————. *Jan Compagnie in Japan, 1600-1850.* The Hague: Martinus Nijhoff, 1950.

Brandt, Maximilian Scipio von. *Dreiunddreissig Jahre in Ostasiens. Erinnerungen eines deutschen Diplomats.* 3 vols. Leipzig: Georg Wigand, 1906.

Burks, Ardath W. "William Elliot Griffis, class of 1869." *Journal of the Rutgers University Library,* September 1966, *29* (3): 91-100.

Cannon, W. B. Letters. W. B. Cannon archives. Boston, Mass. Harvard University Medical School. Countway Library.

Carro, Jean de. *Letters of Jean de Carro to Alexandre Marcet, 1794-1817.* Edited by Henry E. Sigerist. Supplement to the *Bulletin of the History of Medicine,* 12. Baltimore: The Johns Hopkins Press, 1930.

————. *Histoire de la vaccination en Turque et Grèce et aux Indes Orientales.* Sciences et Arts, 6ᵉ année, t. 18, Genève, 1801.

Chamberlain, Basil H. *Things Japanese.* Revised and enlarged edition. London: Kegan Paul, Trench, Trubner and Co. 1890.

Chang, Richard T. "General Grant's 1879 Visit to Japan." *Monumenta Nipponica,* 1969, *24* (4): 373-92.

Dohi Keizo. *Beiträge zur Geschichte der Syphilis insbesondere über ihren Ursprung und ihre Pathologie in Ostasien.* Tokyo: Verlag von Nankodo, 1923.

Éldridge, Stuart. "The occurrence of internal aneurysm in European residents of Japan." *New York Medical Journal,* 1894, *59:* 165-68.

————. "The present state of medicine in Japan." *Medical News,* 1884, *14:* 112-15.

Encyclopedia Japonica. "Aoki Shuzo." Vol. 1. Tokyo: Shogakukan, 1967, p. 63.

Van Esso, I. "Die medizinischen Beziehungen zwischen Japan und Holland." *Janus,* 1941, *45:* 114-36.

Fox, Grace. *Britain and Japan, 1858-1883.* Oxford: Clarendon Press, 1969.

Fujinami Goichi. *Nihon Eisei-shi.* (History of Japanese Medicine.) Nihon Shinshoin, Showa 17, 1943.

Fujikawa, Y. *Japanese Medicine.* Translated by John Ruhräh. New York: Paul B. Hoeber, 1934.

Geschichte der Deutschen Gesellschaft für Natur- und Völkerkunde Ostasiens, 1873-1933. Tokyo: Kojimachi-ku Hirakawa-cho, 1934.

Gratama, Dr. K. W. Letters written to his brother in the Netherlands, during his stay in Japan, April 1866-May 1871.

Great Britain, *Sessional Papers* (Commons) 64, *7* (1869).

Great Britain, *Sessional Papers* (Lords) 1, *16* (1868-1869); 2, *22* (1870).

Griffis, William Elliot. *Hepburn of Japan and His Wife and Helpmates. A Life of Toil for Christ.* Philadelphia: The Westminster Press, 1913.

_____. *The Mikado's Empire.* 10th ed. 2 vols. New York and London: Hayden & Bros., Publishers, 1903.

_____. *Verbeck of Japan, a citizen of no country: A life story of foundation work inaugurated by Guido Fridolin Verbeck.* New York: Revell Co., 1901.

Griffis, William Elliot, and Byas, Hugh. *Japan: A Comparison.* New York: The Japan Society, 1923.

Hachiro Sato. *A Short Biography of English Doctor "William Willis."* Kagoshima: Kagoshima Prefectural Teachers Association Printing Section, 1968.

Halbertsma, K.T.A. "De Beteeknis van de Hollandsche Geneeskunde voor Japan in haar historische Ontwikkeling." *Bijdragen tot de Geschiedenis der Geneeskunde,* 1941, *21:* 106-10.

Hardy, Arthur Sherburne. *The Life and Letters of Joseph Hardy Neesima.* Boston and New York: Houghton Mifflin & Co., 1891.

Harris, Townsend. *The Complete Journal of Townsend Harris.* New York: Doubleday Doran & Co., Inc., 1930.

Hepburn, J. C. *Japan Letters.* United Presbyterian Mission Library, New York.

Hervorragende Tropenärzte in Wort und Bild. Munich: Verlag der Ärztlichen Rundschau, 1932.

Hilgendorf, Franz Martin. Papers, in *Catalogue of Scientific Papers (1800-1900).* 19 vols. London: Royal Society of London, 1867-1925.

Hoffmann, Theodor. "Die Heilkunde in Japan und japanische Ärzte." *Mitteilungen der Deutschen Gesellschaft für Natur- und Völkerkunde Ostasiens,* 1873, *1* (1): 23-25; *1* (4): 9-20.

Hyrtl, Joseph. *Lehrbuch der Anatomie des Menschen mit Rücksicht auf physiologische Begrundung und praktische Anwendung.* 20th ed. Vienna: Wilhelm Braunmüller, 1889.

Irisawa Naika Dosokai, ed. and pub. *Irisawa Sensei no Enzetsu to Bunsho.* Tokyo: Kokuseido, 1932.

Isei Hyakunen-shi. (One Hundred Years of Medical Law.) Koseisho: Imukyoku, 1976.

Ishibashi Choei and Ogawa Teizo. *O-yatoi Gaikokujin-Igaku.* Tokyo: Kajima Kenkyusho Shuppankai, 1969.

Ishihara Akira et al. *Kango Shi.* Tokyo: Igaku Shoin Ltd. Co., 1971.

Jones, Hazel J. "Bakumatsu Foreign Employees." *Monumenta Nipponica,* 1969, 24 (3): 305-27.

————. "The Formulation of the Meiji Government Policy toward the Employment of Foreigners." *Monumenta Nipponica,* 1968, *23* (1-2): 9-30.

Kaempfer, Engelbert. *The History of Japan.* Translated by J. G. Scheuchzer. 2 vols. London, 1727.

Katsuya Narita. *Systems of Higher Education: Japan.* New York: International Council for Educational Development, 1978.

Kawakami Takeshi. *Gendai Nihon no Kyoshi.* Tokyo: Keiso Shobo, 1965.

Kawamata Kenji. *Igeka no rekishi.* Tokyo: Igaku Tosho Publishing Company, 1971.

Keen, W. W., M. D. "On Medical-Missionary Work: with Some Notes on the Condition of Medicine in Japan." *Transactions of the College of Physicians of Philadelphia.* 3rd series, vol. 4. Philadelphia, Pa., 1879.

Keene, Donald. *The Japanese Discovery of Europe, 1720-1830.* Revised edition. Stanford, California: Stanford University Press, 1969.

Kleiweg de Zwaan, J. P. *Völkerkundliches und Geschichtliches über die Heilkunde der Chinesen ünd Japaner mit Besonderer Berücksichtigung Holländischer Einflüsse.* Haarlem: De Erven Loosjes, 1917.

Koichi Uchiyama, M.D. "An Outline of the Historical Development of Physiology in Japan." *Nihon University Journal of Medicine,* December 1961, *3* (4): 1-27.

Latourette, K. S. *A History of Christian Missions in China.* London: Society for Promoting Christian Knowledge, 1929.

Laures, Johannes, S. J. *Kirishitan Bunko.* Tokyo: Sophia University, 1957.

Léger, J. N. *Haiti. Her History and Her Detractors.* New York and Washington, D. C.: The Neale Publishing Co., 1907.

Leyburn, James G. *The Haitian People.* New Haven, Conn.: Yale University Press, 1941.

Mac Lean, J. "The Introduction of Books and Scientific Instruments into Japan, 1712-1854." *Japanese Studies in the History of Science,* 1974, *13:* 9-68.

————. "The Significance of Jan Karel van den Broek (1814-1865) for the Introduction of Western Technology into Japan." *Japanese Studies in the History of Science,* 1977, *16:* 69-90.

McNaught, George K. *See* Robbins, Howard C.

Manson-Bahr, Philip H., and Alcock, A. *The Life of Sir Patrick Manson.* London, Toronto, Melbourne, and Sydney: Cassell & Co. Ltd., 1927.

Van Meerdervoort, J.L.C. Pompe. *Doctor on Desima. Selected Chapters from JHR J. L. C. Pompe van Meerdervoort's "Vijf Jaren in Japan" (1857-1863).* Translated and annotated by Elizabeth P. Wittermans and John Z. Bowers, M. D. Tokyo: Sophia University, 1970.

Meissner, Kurt. *Deutsche in Japan, 1639-1939.* Stuttgart, Berlin: Deutsche Verlags-Anstalt, 1940.

————. "Die Deutschen in Yokohama (Alt-Yokohama)." *Deutsche Gesellschaft für Natur- und Völkerkunde Ostasiens.* Tokyo, 1956.

Mitford, A. B. *Tales of Old Japan.* New York and London: Macmillan & Co., 1893.

Miura, K. "Aus der japanischen Physiognomik." *Mitteilungen der Deutschen Gesellschaft für Natur- und Völkerkunde Ostasiens,* 1902-1903, *9* (1): 7-15.

Miyake, B. "Über die japanische Geburtshelfe." *Mitteilungen der Deutschen Gesellschaft für Natur- und Völkerkunde Ostasiens,* September 1874, *5:* 21-27; September 1875, *8:* 9-13; January 1876, *10:* 9-16.

Mohnike, Otto. "Aanteekeningen over de Geneeskunde der Japanezen." *Geneeskunde Tijdschrift von Nederland-Indie,* 1853, *1:* 198-361.

_____. *Nieuw Nederlandsch Biographisch Woordenboek.* Edited by Dr. P. C. Molhuysen and Dr. F.K.H. Kossmann (with the assistance of Tal van Geleerden). 2 vols. Leiden: A. W. Sijthoff Suitgevers-Maatschaapij N. V., 1937.

_____. Personal Communication from Jansen van Hoof, M.C.J.C. The Hague: Algemeen Rijksarchief's-Gravenhage, 1979.

_____. "Volksaberglauben. Legenden und Ueberlieferungen der Japaner," *Globus,* 1872, 21.

Mueller, Benjamin Karl Leopold. "Tokio-Igaku. Skizzen und Erinnerungen aus der Zeit des geistigen Umschwungs in Japan, 1871-1876." *Deutsche Rundschau,* 1888, *57:* 312-459.

Murdoch, James. *A History of Japan. Vol. III. The Tokugawa Epoch, 1652-1868.* Revised and edited by Joseph H. Longford. London: Kegan Paul, Trench, Trubner and Co., 1926.

Neue Deutsche Biographie, "Max von Brandt." vol. 2. Berlin: Duncker & Humboldt, 1955.

Nihon Igaku Hyakunen-shi. Tokyo: Rinsho Igaku-sha, 1957.

Nishi Seiho, M. D., and Ryoozi Ura, M. D., "The Institute of Anatomy, Imperial University of Japan." *Methods and Problems of Medical Education,* 16th series. New York: The Rockefeller Foundation, 1930, pp. 123-30.

Numata Jiro. *Bakumatsu Yogakushi.* Tokyo: Tokoshoin, 1950.

Ogata Masanori. "Untersuchungen über die Etiologie der *Kak'ke." Ärztliches Intelligenzblatt,* 1885, *32:* 683-86.

Ogata Tomio, ed. *Rangaku to Nihon Bunka.* (*Rangaku* and Japanese Culture.) Report of Symposium on the Historical Relations between the Netherlands and Japan, 7-13 September 1969. Tokyo: Tokyo Daigaku Shuppan-kai, 1971.

Ogawa Teizo. *See also* Ishibashi Choei.

Ogawa Teizo. *Juntendo no Rekishi.* (History of Juntendo.) *Juntendo Soritsu 125 Shunen Kinen Koen.* (Lecture at the 125th Anniversary of Juntendo.). Tokyo, May 21, 1963.

_____, ed. *Tokyo Daigaku Igakubu Hyakunenshi, 1858-1958.* Tokyo: Tokyo Daigaku Igakubu. Soritsu Hyakunen. Kinenkai, 1967.

Ohtani F., M. D. *One Hundred Years of Health Progress in Japan.* (International Medical Foundation of Japan.) Tokyo: Taihei Printing Co., 1971.

Otori Ranzaburo "Rankan Nisshi no Ishigaku teki Kenkyu." ("Medico-historical Studies of Japanese Dagregister, *Nihon Igakushi Kyokai."*) *Journal of the Japan Society of Medical History,* 1962, *10* (1): 11-16.

Pagel, J., ed. *Biographisches Lexikon hervorragenden Ärzte des neunzehnten Jahrhunderts.* Berlin and Vienna: Urban and Schwarzenberg, 1901.

Parsons, Robert P. *History of Haitian Medicine.* New York: Paul B. Hoeber, Inc., 1930.

Peking Union Medical College. *Addresses and Papers, Dedication Ceremonies, and Medical Conference. Peking Union Medical College,* 15-22 September 1921. Concord, N. H.: Rumford Press, 1922.

Refardt, Otto. "Die Deutschen in Kobe." *Mitteilungen der Deutschen Gesellschaft für Natur- und Völkerkunde Ostasiens.* Hamburg and Wiesbaden: Kommissionsverlag Otto Harassowitz, 1868.

Reischauer, Edwin O. *Japan Past and Present.* 2nd ed. Tokyo, Japan, and Rutland, Vermont: Charles E. Tuttle Company, 1952.

————. *Japan: The Story of a Nation.* New York: Alfred A. Knopf, Inc., 1970.

Richards, Linda. "Nursing progress in Japan." *American Journal of Nursing,* April 1902, *2:* 491-94.

Richards, Melinda. *Reminiscences of Melinda Richards, America's First Trained Nurse.* Boston: Whitcomb and Burrows, 1911.

Ride, Lindsay. *Robert Morrison. The Scholar and the Man.* Hong Kong: Hong Kong University Press, 1957.

Robbins, Howard C., and McNaught, George K. *Dr. Rudolf Bolling Teussler. An Adventure in Christianity.* New York: Charles Scribner's Sons, 1942.

Roessingh, M.P.H. *Het Archief van den Nederlandse Factorij in Japan.* (The Archive of the Dutch Factory in Japan (1609-1860). The Hague: Algemeen Rijksarchief, 1964.

————. "Dutch relations with the Philippines, c. 1600-1800. A survey of sources in the General State Archives, The Hague, Netherlands." *Southeast Asian Archives,* July 1909, *2:* 88-103.

Römer, L.S.A.M. von. *Historische Schetsen. Een Inleiding tot het Vierde Congres der Far Eastern Association of Tropical Medicine.* Batavia: Javasche Boekhandel en Drukkerij, 1921.

Rosner, Erhard. "Die Rezeption der westlichen Medizin im Rahmen der Modernisierung Japans zur Meiji-Zeit (1868-1912)." *Medizin, Naturwissenschaft, Technik und das Zweite Kaiserreich.* Vorträge eines Kongresses von 6. bis 11. September 1973 in Bad Nauheim. Göttingen: Vandenhoeck und Ruprecht, 1977.

Rundall, Thomas, ed. *Memorials of the Empire of Japon in the XVI and XVII Centuries.* London: Hakluyt Society, 1850.

Rutgers University. The Griffis Collection. "Education in Japan." *College Courant,* 28 February 1874.

Sansom, G. B. *The Western World and Japan.* New York: Alfred Knopf, 1962.

Satow, Sir Ernest. *A Diplomat in Japan.* London: Seeley & Co. Ltd., 1921.

Scheube, Heinrich Botho. "The Bear Cult and Bear Festivals of the Ainu with Several Remarks about their Dances," *Mitteilungen der Deutschen Gesellschaft für Natur- und Völkerkunde Ostasiens* 21 (1880): 44-52.

————. *Die Ainos.* Yokohama. 1882.

————. "Die japanische *Kak'ke,*" *Mitteilungen der Deutschen Gesellschaft für Natur- und Völkerkunde Ostasiens,* 1880, *3* (28): 170-74.

Schottlander, Felix. *Leben und Werken eines deutschen Arztes in Japan.* Stuttgart: Ausland und Heimat Verlag A. G., 1928.

Schoute, D. *De Geneeskunde in den Dienst der Oost-Indisch Compagnie in Neder-landsch-Indië.* Amsterdam: J. H. DeBussey, 1929.

_____. *Occidental Therapeutics in the Netherlands East Indies during Three Centuries of Netherlands Settlement (1600-1800).* Batavia: Publication of the Netherlands Indies Public Health Service, 1937.

Schultze, Emma and Wilhelm. Letters.

Schultze, Walter Hans. *Ein Lebensbild meines Vaters, Dr. Wilhelm Schultze (1840-1924).* Braunschweig, 1956.

Shimizu Totaro. "Dr. A.J.C. Geerts (1843-1883), a Dutch Pharmacist in Japan." *Yakkyoku, Journal of Practical Pharmacy,* September 1964, *9:* 107-11.

Siddall, J. B. "Surgical Experiences in Military Hospitals in Japan." *St. Thomas's Hospital Reports,* 1914, *5:* 85-112.

Siebold, Alexander von. *Japan's Accession to the Comity of Nations.* Translated by Charles Lowe. London: Kegan Paul, Trench, Trubner & Co. Ltd., 1901.

Simmons, D. B. Letter from Mrs. E. Conklin to W. E. Griffis, 20 November 1911. Rutgers. The State University. Griffis Collection.

_____. "Medical and Sanitary Notes on the Foreign Settlements of Eastern and Southern Asia." *Medical Record,* 1881, *19:* 386-88.

_____. "Medical Notes on Eastern and Southern Asia." *Medical Record,* 1882, *21:* 248-49.

_____. "Medical Practice in Japan, Old and New." *Medical Record,* 1881, *19:* 204-6

_____. "The Diseases of Japan." *Medical Record,* 1881, *19:* 90-92.

Smith, George. *Ten Weeks in Japan.* London: Longman, Green, Longman, and Roberts, 1861.

Tadashi Inoue. *Introduction and Generalization of Jennerian Vaccination in Japan. Rangaku to Nihon Bunka.* Ogata Tomio, ed. Tokyo Daigaku Shuppan-Kai, 1970.

Tanaka Yukichi. *Meiji Taisho Nihon Igaku Shi.* (History of Japanese Medicine in the Meiji-Taisho Eras.) Tokyo, 1927.

Townsend, William John. *Robert Morrison. The Pioneer of Chinese Missions.* London: S. W. Partridge & Co., 1892.

Vallery-Radot, René. *The Life of Pasteur.* Translated by R. L. Devonshire. New York: Doubleday, Page & Company, 1927.

Verbeck, Rev. G. F. "Early Mission Days in Japan." *Japan Advertiser,* 30 October 1926.

Vescovi, Gerhard. *Erwin Baelz: Wegbereiter der japanischen Medizin.* Stuttgart: A. W. Gentner Verlag, 1972.

De Waart, A. "Medical education in the Dutch East Indies." *Addresses and Papers, Dedication Ceremonies and Medical Conference, Peking Union Medical College.* Peking, 1922.

Wagenseil, F. "Die drei ersten unter europäischem (holländischem) Einfluss ent-standenen japanischen Anatomiebücher." *Sudhoffs Archiv für Geschichte der Medizin und der Naturwissenschaften,* 1959, *43:* 61-85.

Wernich, A.L.A. "Über Ausbreitung und Bedeutung der neuen Culturbestrebungen in Japan." *Deutsche Zeit- und Streitfragen,* 1877, *6* (93).

_____. "Uber die Fortschritte der modernen Medizin in Japan." *Berliner*

Klinische Wochenschrift, 1875, *12:* 447, 474, 590, 655, 667; 1876, *13:* 107.

Whitney, Willis Norton. "Notes on the History of Medical Progress in Japan." *Transactions of the Asiatic Society of Japan,* 1885, *12:* 245-467.

Williams, Frederick Wells. *The Life and Letters of Samuel Wells Williams, LL. D., Missionary, Diplomatist, and Sinologue.* New York and London: G. P. Putnam's Sons, The Knickerbocker Press, 1889.

Willis, William. Obituary notices. *Lancet,* 1894, *i:* 507-8; *British Medical Journal,* 24 February 1894, *i:* 441.

_____. "Reports of journeys in China and Japan." Great Britain, *Sessional Papers* (Lords) 1, 16 (1868-1869).

_____. "Correspondence respecting Diplomatic and Consular Expeditions in China, Japan, and Siam." Ibid. 2, 22 (1870).

Wohl, Herbert. "James Curtis Hepburn, M. D. 1815-1911 (Hepburn of Japan)." *New England Journal of Medicine,* December 3, 1970, *283:* 1271-74.

Wong, K. Chimin, and Wu Lien-teh. *History of Chinese Medicine.* Tientsin: Tientsin Press, 1934.

Wunsch, Richard. M. D. *Artzt in Ostasien.* Edited by Gertrud Claussen-Wunsch. Büsingen-Hochrhein: Krämer Verlag, 1976.

Index

169